Backache

What you need to know

DR DAVID DELVIN

PRESS

Dedicated to Christine – whose massage has helped me enormously.

First published in Great Britain in 2009
Sheldon Press
36 Causton Street
London SW1P 4ST

British Library Cataloguing-in-Publication Data
A catalogue record for this book is available from the British Library

ISBN 978–1–84709–060–7

1 3 5 7 9 10 8 6 4 2

Typeset by Fakenham Photosetting Ltd, Fakenham, Norfolk
Printed in Great Britain by Ashford Colour Press

Produced on paper from sustainable forests

Contents

Acknowledgements

I should like to thank all those who have helped with my researches into backache over the last 35 years, and indeed with this book. They include:

The late Dr James Cyriax, MD, MRCP
Dr Tom Smith, MB, Dip Pharm Med RCP
Mr James MacCabe, FRCS Ed.
Ralph Hammond
Ben Cull, DO
Peter Blagrave, DO
Dr Peter Dixon, DC
Tim Hutchful, DC
Sara Bailey
Ms Christine Webber, LNCP, MNCH

Also ... a number of osteopaths and chiropractors, many physiotherapists ... and all those who have consulted me with back pain.

However, any mistakes in this book are entirely my own responsibility.

Introduction

When a GP has a full waiting room, it usually contains two or three men and women with backache. In fact, the number of people off work each day in the UK because of back pain would fill London's new Olympic stadium.

The UK's national back pain charity, BackCare, estimates that in industrialized countries roughly 80 per cent of the population will experience backache at some stage in their lives.

Recently, the British Chiropractic Association claimed that at any given moment, one in three of us has backache. I have a feeling that this figure might be a slight over-estimate, but it does give support to my view that this is one of the most common afflictions of the human race.

Where backache is concerned, I speak from personal experience. Although I'm a doctor, I have had an awful lot of back trouble myself. Happily, I have learned how to defeat it.

And, during the last 35 years or so, I have tried out for myself most of the available treatments for backache – including the 'orthodox' ones, such as medication, injections, physiotherapy and surgery, and the so-called 'alternative' ones, such as osteopathy, chiropractic, acupuncture and the Alexander technique – and even hanging upside-down …

In this book, I'm going to tell you about all the treatments that could help your backache, and I'll also be explaining how you can avoid future attacks of pain.

One word of warning: there are a lot of different schools of thought with regard to the treatment of backache, as you will discover in these pages. They do compete with one another, and sometimes criticize one another. And my experience has been that some individuals make sweeping and unscientific statements in order to bolster their own theories or practices.

So if a practitioner tells you something about your case that seems rather improbable, don't hesitate to ask him or her: 'What is the evidence for that, please?' If it isn't forthcoming, seek another opinion.

Please read on – and good luck!

Dr David Delvin

Publisher's note: This book is not intended to replace advice from your GP. Do consult your doctor if you are experiencing symptoms with which you feel you need help.

1

Why backache is so common – and how to prevent it

So pain in the back is one of the most common afflictions of man – and woman. Why?

Well, it's mainly because we put our backs through all sorts of stresses and strains that the human spine just isn't equipped to cope with. I'm talking about things like:

- lifting heavy weights;
- bending over – especially to pick things up off the floor;
- sitting – especially on uncomfortable chairs;
- twisting round – especially in the car;
- suddenly leaping out of bed without supporting your weight on your arms;
- being overweight – which increases the work the spine has to do.

The stresses on your back

Why can't our backs cope with all these things? It's because the poor, battered old human back is an enormously complicated structure. As we'll see in the next chapter, your spine is made up of more than 30 irregularly shaped bones, linked to one another by many quite complex joints. Between these bones are little discs of cartilage, which are so positioned that they can all too easily bulge out and press on a nerve root.

The whole spine is surrounded by dozens of muscles and ligaments; and around it run a multitude of nerves and blood vessels. Furthermore, going down through a tunnel in the centre of your spine there is the spinal cord – the big communications channel of your body.

Please imagine that you somehow or other managed to build a model of all this – say, out of Meccano or Lego. Inevitably, it would be an unwieldy and rather delicate structure. Now imagine furthermore that you got hold of this 'model', and bent or twisted it in various directions.

What would happen? Well, something would give way of course. There would be a crack or a twang, and one of the components would burst apart from another.

That's roughly what happens when we put our backs through the various stresses of daily life. We bend over, or we twist round, or we grab awkwardly at an object, and – ping! – something goes. Result: pain.

Incidentally, it's often said that it's only humans, and other 'walking upright' animals, that get back trouble. That is not quite right. For instance, disc problems have been found in the spines of dinosaurs.

However, it is true that being upright creatures, people are forced to put a lot of strains on the back. Unlike us, dogs and cats do not have to bend over in order to reach things on the ground. Nor do they lift heavy weights with their front paws, as we do. Neither do they sit in badly designed seats, or drive cars! As a result, cats and dogs don't get backache as much as humans do – or so my veterinary colleagues tell me.

So humankind is a bit stuck with an awkward, complex, vertical structure called 'the back', and we have to do some fairly tricky manoeuvres with it.

Nevertheless, it is possible to go through life treating your back sensibly, so as to minimize the strains on it. This chapter will show you how.

Let's now have a look at the factors that are likely to cause backache, and see what can be done about them.

Lifting the wrong way

If I had to pick one thing, above all others, that results in humans getting back pain, it would be lifting. If you lift things in the wrong way, that puts a huge strain on your back. And, alas, most people lift things in the wrong way.

When I was young, I felt I could lift almost anything – and could do it any old how. I used to thoughtlessly pick up heavy weights off the floor. I used to lift up my little daughter, and sweep her up over my head. I would go to the gym, casually grasp a bar-bell and jerk it up into the air. When playing with my children, I'd show off by lifting big boulders from a mountainside, and throwing them about.

Eventually, of course, I got a 'slipped disc' – and that certainly taught me a lesson about the folly of lifting things in the wrong way.

So what *is* 'the wrong way'? Have a look at the man in Figure 1.1.

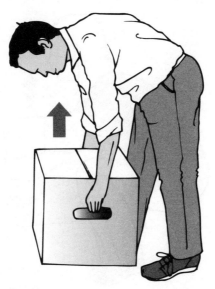

Figure 1.1 Lifting badly

As you see, he is about to lift a box off the floor. He's reaching for it by bending his back forwards. His knees are straight. So when he tries to lift the box, he'll have to do it entirely with his back. He'll straighten up, putting immense strain on his spine. This is a recipe for disaster.

He may get away with this kind of lifting 20, 30 or even 50 times – but the odds are that eventually something will give. Result: severe backache.

Lifting the right way

Then what is the *right* way to lift? Have a look at the woman in Figure 1.2.

You'll observe that in order to lift her box off the floor, she isn't bending her back. Instead, she has kept it straight. To get down low enough to pick up the box, she has bent her knees.

I can't over-emphasize the message that this is the correct way to lift things off the floor. Always bend your knees, and not your back. Whether you're picking up a heavy load at work, or lifting your toddler, or grabbing a shopping bag from the floor, the principle is the same: *use your knees, not your spine.*

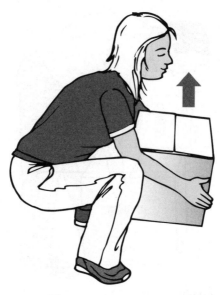

Figure 1.2 Lifting correctly

By adopting this simple axiom, you can save yourself an awful lot of back trouble. Now you might say, 'But isn't this just transferring the strain to the knees?'

That's true. But the fact is that your knees are far better equipped for the strain of lifting than your back is. Admittedly, people often get knee injuries, and even arthritis of the knee. But, in general, these problems aren't caused by lifting. Your knee joints are well able to withstand what for them is the relatively minor stress of lifting up a handbag or a laptop from the floor. In contrast, your back is highly likely to go badly wrong if you use it to lift things by straightening it.

Keeping weights close to your body

Up till now, we've been talking about lifting objects off the floor. But you can also strain your back by lifting things off tables, desks or shelves and carrying them. Have a look at the man in Figure 1.3.

He is trying to carry a large box by holding it at arms' length. This is not at all wise. If you're lifting any significant weight, *you should keep it as close as possible to your body*. That makes life easier – and the strain on your back much less.

You may be interested to know that this is an old judo principle. All those learning judo are taught that it is much simpler to pick up

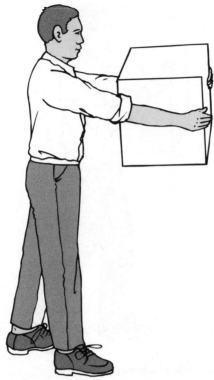

Figure 1.3 Carrying a load badly

and throw an opponent if you can hold him tight against your body – rather than struggling to lift him up while holding him half a metre or so away from you.

Similarly, if you look at the man in Figure 1.4, you'll see the best way of lifting and carrying a heavy box – the object is close to his body. You'll find it much easier to lift, and there will be less strain on your spine.

Bending the wrong way

Another activity that causes back trouble is bending – even if no lifting is involved. The human spine really isn't equipped for doing things like bending forward and 'touching your toes'. Nor does it like excessive sideways or backward bending.

So if you keep bending over – whether it is in your job, round the house, or maybe in some sporting activity – there is quite a chance that

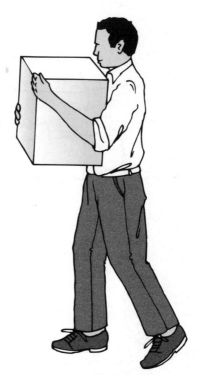

Figure 1.4 Carrying a load correctly

something will 'go' in your spinal area, so that you will be left with a nasty backache.

To illustrate this point, look at Figure 1.5.

The golfer in Figure 1.5 is bending right over to tee up his ball, thus putting immense strain on his spine. I forecast that before too long, he'll be in big trouble.

Bending the right way

In contrast, look at the tennis player in Figure 1.6.

She is picking up a ball from the court. But, very sensibly, instead of bending her spine right over, she has thrown out a leg behind her, thus ensuring that her spine stays fairly straight. Somehow, I don't think *she'll* be getting backache tonight.

But it's not just bending all the way down to the ground that results in backache. Just bending a couple of feet forwards can cause problems, if you're not careful.

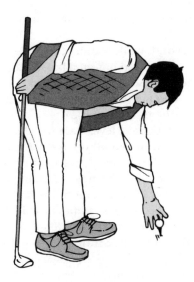

Figure 1.5 Golfer bending over badly

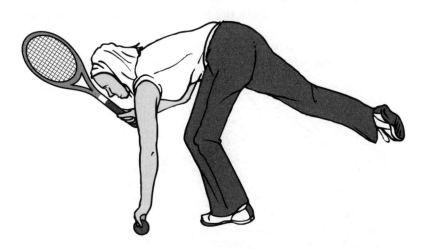

Figure 1.6 Tennis player bending correctly

For instance, many people work at tables or desks. If you're sitting down, that's fine. But consider the situation of the woman in Figure 1.7.

She is an architect and, while standing up, she is working on drawings and papers that are spread out on a broad office table. Every time she bends forward to reach something on the far side of the table, she is putting massive stress on her lumbar spine and on her sacro-iliac joints (more about them in the next chapter).

On a slightly more mundane level, I am the chief 'table-layer' in our house. I really enjoy putting out all the items for a nice dinner party, with lots of gleaming cutlery, wine glasses and candles. However, I realized a few years ago that doing this while standing upright was lunacy. The strain on my spine as I leaned over to the far side of the table was really giving me 'gyp'. So, after a couple of episodes of quite severe sacro-iliac pain, I changed my whole technique for table-laying. These days I actually lay the table while sitting down – it's easy, comfortable and safe.

A few more tips about bending:

- Does the arrangement of your kitchen make everyone bend down a lot? For instance, are the saucepans stored just a couple of feet off the ground? If so, consider rearranging things, so that objects that you need frequently are stashed at a convenient height – say a metre, or 1.5 metres, above the ground. That way, you'll do much less bending.
- Similarly, if you have an office or a study, make sure that the stuff you most often reach for (files, reference books, pads of paper,

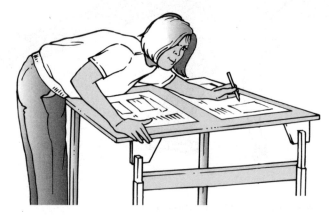

Figure 1.7 Architect leaning forward awkwardly over a table

envelopes, whatever) is kept at waist-height or higher, so that you don't have to keep bending to reach them.

- Consider having the 'on-off' for your computer at a reasonable height. Very often, these little switches are somewhere down near the floor, making it really awkward to reach them.
- If you're fitting out a new house or flat, consider having the power-points at, say, hip-height instead of the usual position, just above the skirting-board. That way, you'll bend much less.
- Remember the wise words of comedian Ronnie Corbett, who once said: 'These days, when I bend over to get something, I have a look round and ask myself if there's anything else I can do *while I'm down here* ...'

Sitting badly and sitting well

A lot of backache is caused by sitting in ways that throw the bones of the spine out of alignment. That's why it's so often the case that people stand up from chairs with a groan, and clutch their lower backs.

There are two main things that can cause problems: the sitter's posture, and the actual chair.

Let's begin by looking at posture. Regrettably, many of us sit in a way that throws an awful lot of stress on the spine. I know that for years and years *I* did this, and it contributed to my many episodes of back pain. These days, I've learnt my lesson.

The two most common mistakes in posture are shown in Figure 1.8.

The woman on the left is sitting slouched in her chair, with her bottom far away from the back of the seat. This means that there's no support for her lumbar spine, which is the bit just above her buttocks. Many people do this – and end up with what is sometimes called lumbago, a word that actually just means 'pain in the lumbar area'.

The man sitting in the middle isn't doing too well either. As you see, he's got his shoulders slumped forward, so that the upper part of his back isn't supported by the chair. If he goes on sitting like this, he will very likely run into painful problems with his upper spine.

However, the person on the right is sitting well. His posture is so good that even sitting in a chair for hours isn't likely to give him backache.

If you think that *you* have problems with posture, it would be well worth your while having some sessions with an 'Alexander technique' therapist (see Chapter 11).

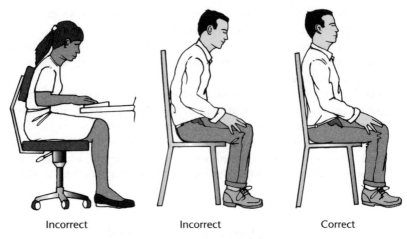

| Incorrect | Incorrect | Correct |

Figure 1.8 Sitting correctly and incorrectly

So, we can do a lot to avoid backache by always sitting sensibly. But, as I mentioned, there's an additional problem: the shape of the chair or seat that you're using.

Seating

Many of those with back pain are well aware that there are certain chairs that bring on pain, so you obviously need to avoid these at all costs. At work, if you're given a chair that causes you backache, then you really *must* insist on having it changed. No reasonable employer would refuse such a request. After all, if he does refuse and if you damage your back as a result, he might get sued ...

In practice, it's mainly seating at work that causes back problems. At home, people generally seem to manage to pick themselves chairs that are comfortable, ones that don't cause aches and pains around the spine.

When in a shop buying a chair, try to find one that will fit snugly to the curve of your lower back, and give you a reasonable amount of support. Sit on it for a little while before deciding to make your purchase. If it hurts you, don't buy it.

These days, a lot of people buy chairs and other furniture via the internet or from catalogues. I advise against this. If you're going to sit on something for the next 25 years, you really do need to try it out first.

One good thing is that the design of seating has improved quite a lot in the last couple of decades. Chair and sofa designers are now well aware that if they don't provide support for the 'sitter's' spine, that's going to lead to backache.

Car seats

Unfortunately, car seats are a major cause of back pain – although I must admit that the design of them seems to have improved significantly in recent years. Nevertheless, a lot of people come into my consulting room and say 'The pain's worse after I've been sitting in the car for an hour, doc.'

If that happens to *you*, then the sane thing to do is to change your car. And when you're buying a new vehicle, I strongly suggest that you spend ten minutes or so sitting in the front seat before you decide to purchase. Since these days we spend such a lot of our time at the wheel (or in the passenger seat), it's vital to ensure that the seating is OK.

Other seats

You also need to be wary of airline seats and train seats. Airline seating has improved a bit in recent times, but you may find that a long flight gives you backache – particularly if you're flying on one of the budget airlines whose seats are ludicrously close together.

The design of train seats is often pretty poor, particularly in the UK, where sadly it is commonplace for broken seating to be left unrepaired by the rail company.

Cinema seats don't seem to give people all that much trouble these days, especially as the big multiplex chains seem to have realized that it pays to give customers a bit of space and comfort.

But theatre seats – at least in the UK – are often appallingly bad for the back. Many older theatres have a cramped seating plan that may have been acceptable to very small Victorians, but that gives totally inadequate room for a tall or even medium-height person. Many is the time I've limped out of a London theatre, ruefully rubbing the small of my back. (*Tip*: it might be a good idea to book yourself a seat on the end of a row, so that you can stretch out more.)

If you're prone to back pain, then on planes and trains, and in cinemas and theatres, it may be worthwhile taking a small cushion with you to jam in behind the lumbar area of your spine.

Back aids (supports)

A useful alternative are the 'back supports' manufactured by many companies. These are little purpose-designed cushions, pads or plates that are designed to fit into the curve of the lumbar area. Some of them are inflatable, so you can pump them up to whatever size is comfortable for you. At the time of writing, you can buy them for between £19 and £65.

I am definitely *not* recommending any particular brand, but well-known ones in the UK include:

- Posture Curve;
- LumbarMate;
- MedAir Inflatable;
- Putnam – various models;
- MEDesign Back Friend;
- Obusforme Backrest Support.

You can buy all of the above via the internet. However, I think it's better to go to a specialist back-pain shop or a large pharmacy, so you can 'try before you buy'.

Twisting

One thing to avoid at all costs is putting excessive strain on your back by *twisting*. Twisting round creates dangerous stresses in your spine, especially if you bend at the same time.

These days, the most common example of this is what happens when people are sitting in the front seat of a car. They twist right round to see what's coming behind, instead of using all the mirrors. Or they decide that they want to get something from the back seat. So they twist their poor old spines through well over 90 degrees, and then bend over sideways in an effort to grab whatever it is they're after. All too often, the result is that they feel something 'go' – and then get back pain for the next few days or weeks.

So, if you can't easily reach something that's on the back seat of your car, *leave it alone*. If it's really necessary to have it, then stop the car, get out, and stand outside before you reach in and grasp it.

Incidentally, I have found that (if you can afford it) a four-door car makes life a lot easier for those who are prone to back pain. While standing outside of it, you can get things out of the back without having to fight your way past the front seat. And obviously, it makes getting into the rear of the car (to sit on the back seat) much simpler, and much less likely to put strain on your spine.

Also, be very wary of twisting your back as you get out of bed. If you're prone to backache, you should use your arms to get yourself into an upright position. Then swing your legs over the edge of the bed, so that your feet are on or near the ground. Finally, push down with your hands in order to stand up.

Being overweight

Alas, there is little doubt that carrying excess weight puts a strain on your spine, and is quite likely to lead to backache. I say 'Alas' because the fact is that I myself have always carried too many pounds! Yes, I'm trying to do something about it …

It is true that plenty of slim people also get back problems. But pain in the back is more likely to strike those who are carrying a 'spare tyre'. This is simply because the spine is a delicate and vulnerable structure – a structure that is easily pulled 'out of true' by having excess weight hung on it.

So if you are overweight and can slim down a bit, you will do your back a lot of good.

Summing up

Backache can happen out of the blue, but very often it's caused by factors that you can do something about.

These factors include lifting, bending, sitting awkwardly, twisting, and being overweight. If you keep getting back pain, it's worth thinking about these things, and seeing what you can do about them.

In the next chapter, we'll take a look at the structures that make up your back – and what can go wrong with them.

2

The structure of your back – and why it hurts

If you get a lot of backache, it's well worth making an effort to understand the structure of your back, and in particular your spine.

Surprisingly, few people have much knowledge of this important area of the body. Certainly, in the UK most of us were never taught anything about it at school – even if we did Human Biology at GCSE.

For example, it's very rare for women or men who come into my consulting room to have heard of the sacro-iliac joint – which is often the cause of back pain. Things are a bit different in the USA and some other countries, where it's commonplace to hear people say: 'Gee, doc, I'm having real trouble with my sacro-iliac this week!'

Your spine, spinal column or backbone

So let's run through the basic anatomy of the human back. Have a look at the rear view of the woman in Figure 2.1.

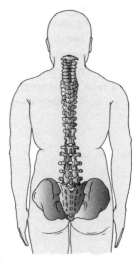

Figure 2.1 The back, showing anatomy of the spine

14

You can see that her spine is composed of a column of small bones, piled on top of each other. It's rather as if you took 30 or so draughts or checkers, and balanced them on one another, in a tower.

This vertical column of bones is called 'the spine' or 'the spinal column' – or, sometimes, 'the backbone'. It runs downwards from the base of the skull to the area between the buttocks. You can feel these little knobbly bones by just running your fingertips up and down the middle of your back.

Each of the bones is called a 'vertebra' – and the plural of 'vertebra' is the word 'vertebrae'. (It's usually pronounced 'ver-tuh-bree'.)

Your ligaments and joints

Obviously, a pile of 30-odd checkers or draughts would soon fall over if they didn't have any support. Well, your backbone *does* have support. In fact, the entire column of bones is all bound together by ligaments.

These are much the same as the sheets of tissue that you'll see holding bones together when you carve a joint of meat. So, it's rather as if that column of draughts or checkers is all kept together by sheets of cling-film wrapped round it.

The only problem with this excellent arrangement is that it's possible for the ligaments to get torn – if we twist or bend our backs too far or too violently. That hurts!

The vertebrae are in contact with many other bones. In fact, there are well over 100 different joints in your back. (A 'joint' is just a place where two bones meet.)

Many of these joints can get wrenched or slightly displaced by excessive twisting or bending motions of the spine. A slight displacement of this kind is called a 'subluxation'. And, once again, it hurts a lot ...

Your facet joints

The vertebrae feel knobbly because they have all sorts of bony projections sticking out from them. You can see what I mean by looking at Figure 2.2.

These projections are very useful, because they provide attachments for a lot of important structures – mainly muscles and ligaments. But, alas, the complexity of all these 'sticky-out' bits is so great that it's very easy for things to go wrong with them.

In particular, you'll see that the vertebra in the diagram has a

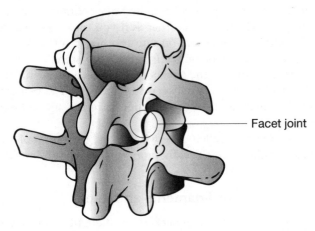

Figure 2.2 Facet joint

projection that goes upwards and touches a projection coming downwards from the bone immediately above.

The area where the two bones meet is called a 'facet joint'. It is made
up of two smooth surfaces, each about as big as a fingernail.

You only have to glance at this joint to see that the opportunities
for something to go wrong with it are very great. Imagine its owner
bending forward or twisting sideways. Anyone can see that it would
be very easy for the lower bone to slip slightly out of position (what
is often called a subluxation) – and to start grinding against the one
above.

I've experienced this numerous times, and I can assure you that it is
extremely painful. It's called 'facet joint syndrome'.

If you happen to live near one of those health shops that have a
skeleton in the window, you can get an even clearer impression of
what happens in facet joint syndrome. Just look at the skeleton, and
imagine what would happen if somebody took hold of that spine in
both hands, and then twisted and bent it. There would be a heck of a
lot of crunching – and many of those little facet joints would be par-
tially dislocated, wouldn't they? Regrettably, that sort of painful event
happens to the human spine very frequently.

Your spinal cord and nerve roots

Now what is the spinal cord? Well, it's a long 'cable' of nerve tissue that runs downwards from your brain to the lower part of your back, as you can see in Figure 2.3.

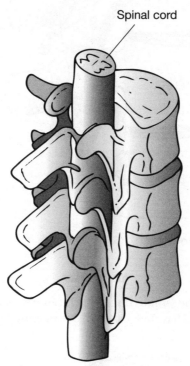

Spinal cord

Figure 2.3 Spinal cord

It is protected by the bones of the spine, because it passes through the middle of each one, as far down as the upper lumbar region. It is the main communications channel of your body, since it carries nearly all the messages from your brain to your arms, legs and trunk.

When you want to move, say, your toe, your brain sends a signal down through the spinal cord, and then on downwards through the nerves that supply the muscles that curl or stretch the toes.

The roots of these nerves come out of your spinal cord, and then emerge from the spine by passing through the tiny spaces that lie between the vertebrae. You can see this arrangement in Figure 2.4.

Regrettably, this rather cramped set-up makes the nerve roots extremely vulnerable to being compressed – especially by discs ...

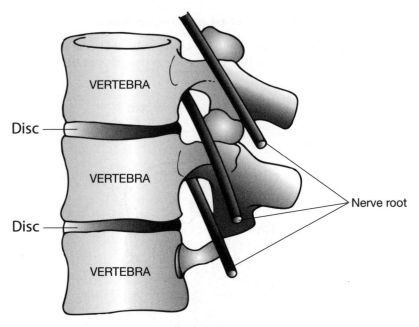

Figure 2.4 Nerve roots

Your discs

Now we come to the famous discs, which cause such a lot of severe back pain. You can see what they look like by studying Figure 2.5.

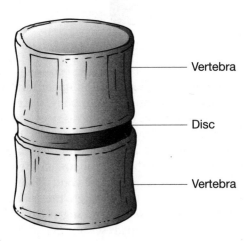

Figure 2.5 Disc

Each disc looks rather like a tiny hamburger, or a miniature ice hockey puck. They're all made of the tough springy material called 'cartilage', which you may know better as 'gristle'.

What do they do? Well, a disc is a shock-absorber. In other words, it cushions the impact that occurs when two of the vertebrae are pushed hard together. This shock-absorption is a very good thing. For example, if you jump off a wall and land on your feet, the discs will cushion the blow, so that your spinal bones don't bash together too violently.

The downside of all this is that the spinal discs are very vulnerable to misuse – that is, excessive lifting, bending or twisting. If a disc is subjected to too much stress, part of it will *bulge* outwards.

You can see what that means by looking at Figure 2.6.

A little bit of disc is bulging out to one side – and it's pressing on a nerve root. This is the infamous 'slipped disc' – though it hasn't really slipped; it's just bulging. But because the bulge is pressing on the root of a nerve, it will give you tremendous pain.

Very often, you will feel this pain in the area of your body that the nerve supplies. Most commonly of all, disc trouble in the lumbar region (i.e. your lower back) will cause you pain running right down to your heel.

Disc problems are dealt with fully in Chapter 10.

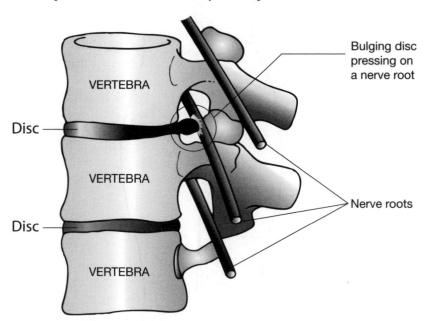

Figure 2.6 Bulging disc, pressing on nerve root

Your sacro-iliac joints

Finally, we come to the sacro-iliac joints (or 'S-I' joints), which are a common source of backache.

In Figure 2.7, you can see that all the weight carried by your spine has to rest on your two iliac bones, which are part of your pelvis. The joint where the sacrum meets your iliac bone is called the sacro-iliac.

The sacro-iliac joint is located just under the little dimple that is seen in many people, right at the top of the buttock. Put your fingertip on this dimple, and you probably will be able to feel your own S-I joint, not far below the skin.

So at this point, two fairly big bones are rubbing against each other. If you put your palms together, and then slide them up and down a few millimetres, you'll get the general idea of what the joint is like.

Most of the time, this S-I joint works just fine. But ... very often it happens that excess bending or lifting makes one side of the joint slip a little too far – and then jam. This is the cause of sacro-iliac pain. As you might expect, it mainly occurs just to the left or right of the lowest part of the spine – near that well-known dimple, in fact.

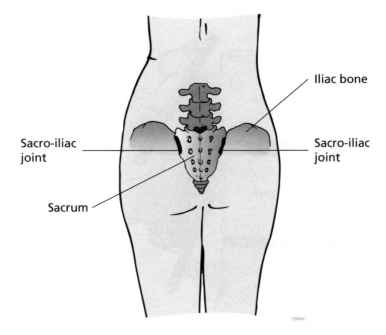

Figure 2.7 Sacro-iliac (S-I) joints

I've had a bit of S-I joint trouble on dozens of occasions in my life. The most recent episode occurred when I bent a little too enthusiastically forwards while strimming the lawn. Ouch! This pain can be quite disabling for a few days or more. One characteristic feature is that it makes it very difficult for you to get up from a chair.

S-I joint difficulties are very well understood by osteopaths and chiropractors. They are good at manipulating the joint, so as to ease the pain and speed recovery. However, in my researches into back pain, I have been a bit surprised to find that some doctors aren't very aware of sacro-iliac joint problems and fail to diagnose the cause of the trouble.

So, if you have an S-I problem, my advice to you is to go and get yourself manipulated by an expert.

Summing up

So you can see that the structure of your back is extraordinarily complicated, and that many things can go wrong with it. Indeed, I reckon it's surprising that we humans don't spend our entire lives suffering from back pain.

3

What causes backache?

In the previous chapter, we looked at the very complex anatomy of your back. But what exactly can go wrong with it? When you get a pain in your back, what could the actual diagnosis be? And why are doctors and other health professionals often a bit reluctant to say exactly what's wrong?

The difficulties of diagnosis

You may be surprised to hear that the diagnosis of the precise cause of a pain in the back is *not* easy at all. The structure of the human back is so very complicated that it is usually quite difficult to state *exactly* what the cause of the pain is.

Also, in most cases there are no lab tests or investigations that would help. People often think that an X-ray would immediately reveal what the cause of their pain is, but in the great majority of cases, that isn't so – because X-rays can only show quite gross abnormalities of the bones. They do not really show up what are called 'soft tissues', like muscles and ligaments.

So it's often very difficult indeed to say with absolute precision what's causing back pain. In fact, if you went to, say, three different doctors and a physiotherapist, plus an osteopath and a chiropractor, it wouldn't be too surprising if you ended up by being given six slightly different diagnoses.

In practice, many GPs tend to avoid giving a really precise diagnosis. Instead, they say something like: 'I can tell you that this isn't serious, and that it should get better soon.' And most of the time they're right.

It was about 30 years ago when I first realized the enormous difficulties of making a pinpoint diagnosis in cases of backache. I had invited one of the world's leading back specialists, the late Dr James Cyriax, to address a meeting of GPs. He was a very clever man, and a good doctor, and I had cause to be grateful to him for the treatment that he gave me.

I introduced the great expert to his audience, and he stood up at a lectern, and began to speak. His first words were: 'Ladies and gentlemen, as you all know, the commonest cause of back pain is a prolapsed [i.e. bulging] disc.'

I was also on the platform, chairing the meeting, and as I looked round the room at the assembled GPs, I observed their jaws dropping with astonishment. You see, from their own general practices, it was perfectly obvious to them that the most common cause of backache was *not* a 'slipped disc'. They knew very well that the majority of those who consulted them had relatively minor – if rather undiagnosable – causes of back trouble, and that most of these people got better within a few weeks.

Interestingly, none of the GPs had the nerve to get up and challenge the famous expert about his rather sweeping statement. And neither did I ...

Later, I realized that the probable explanation for this strange clash of views was fairly simple. At his elegant consulting rooms, the world-renowned specialist saw only people who had relatively *serious* causes of backache – including me, incidentally. Most of these people did indeed have disc lesions.

Brilliant as he was, Dr Cyriax had no real idea that out in the world of general practice there were hordes of people who had brief spells of backache that got better in a fortnight or so, after a bit of rest plus gentle exercise, and perhaps a course of anti-inflammatory pills. Such people never came anywhere near him.

Diagnosis in general practice

So what *does* cause the average person's fairly short-lived backache? If you press a GP, she will probably give you a list of possibilities, which would be something like this:

- minor tears of muscles;
- minor tears of ligaments;
- minor displacements of one of the many dozens of joints in the spine.

The last category would include the two important diagnoses that I mentioned in the last chapter:

- facet joint syndrome;
- sacro-iliac joint syndrome.

But, in general, your GP may well be a bit non-committal with regard to your backache, and just say that it's a minor mechanical problem, which should get better soon.

Osteopathic diagnosis

In contrast, if you asked an osteopath for the most common cause of back pain, he might perhaps talk about 'the osteopathic lesion'. This is a term that was introduced long ago by the founder of osteopathy, Andrew Taylor Still (1828–1917).

What does it mean? Well, if you search the internet you will find all sorts of definitions for it, some of them a trifle vague. Currently, it is often defined as 'the somatic dysfunction' – which I don't think is a tremendously helpful explanation. However, leading UK osteopath Bill Ferguson explains 'the osteopathic lesion' like this: 'An osteopathic lesion is simply a joint in which there is anything from a slight to a total limitation of the normal physiological range of movement.'

That seems pretty fair to me. Certainly, many back pains do seem to be caused by minor derangements (subluxations) of one of the dozens of joints in the spine. And skilled manipulation of these joints will often ease the pain, or sometimes abolish it completely.

There is much more about osteopathy in Chapter 6.

Chiropractic diagnosis

And what would happen if you asked a chiropractor what the causes of back pain are? He would probably agree with leading American chiropractic expert Steven G. Yeomans, who says that they can be divided into three categories:

- very serious but rare causes, like spinal fractures, spinal infections and cancer;
- fairly serious nerve root pains – like those caused by a disc;
- most commonly, mechanical causes.

By 'mechanical causes', chiropractors mean minor injuries and subluxations. (This word is used in different senses by chiropractors and doctors, but roughly speaking it means 'minor joint displacements'.) Like osteopaths, chiropractors believe that these conditions often respond well to manipulation – or, as they call it, 'adjustment'. And they are right.

There is a lot more about chiropractic in Chapter 7.

Medical diagnosis by triage

Nowadays, most medical doctors who are interested in back pain tend to use a similar 'sorting' classification to the one I've just listed. The idea is to decide whether a person who comes in with back pain has:

A something very serious;
B a disc/nerve root problem;
C a minor mechanical derangement.

This system of classifying problems is called 'triage'. People often think that the word means 'dividing into three', but in fact it's just the French for 'sorting'.

So when you come into the surgery and say that you've got backache, your doctor should ask you some questions and then examine you. On the basis of what you've told her, plus her examination, she should be able to make a reasonable assessment of which of the three categories applies to *you*.

Can I just stress that the serious Category 'A' – which includes cancer – is rare. But if you're really worried about that sort of thing, then have a look at Chapter 12.

Category 'B' – in which a disc causes pain by pressing on a nerve root – is much more common. The thing that gives it away is that the pain usually runs down your leg, or occasionally down your arm. You'll find details of this sort of problem in Chapter 10.

Finally, Category 'C' covers the vast majority of cases of back pain – things like muscle and ligament tears, facet joint problems, and sacro-iliac joint trouble. These difficulties can be a terrible nuisance, but they're not going to cripple you, or keep you in agony for the rest of your life. Most of the time, they will get better quite soon, helped by gentle exercise, warmth, sensible amounts of rest, and perhaps anti-inflammatory or pain-killing medication, plus maybe some manipulation. Avoidance of lifting, bending and other stresses to the back is also important.

For fuller details of how you can deal with these annoying but minor mechanical problems of the back, and how they are treated, please see Chapter 4.

Lumbago

The great majority of backaches occur in the lumbar region – that is, the 'small of the back', just above the buttocks. This is because so much spinal movement takes place in that area. Pain in the lumbar zone is still sometimes referred to by the old name 'lumbago'. People often think that this is an actual diagnosis of the cause of their backache, but it isn't. The word 'lumbago' is derived from 'lumbar' and 'ague' (pain), and it just means 'pain low down in the back'.

Summing up

So, to sum up, it's obvious that if you get backache, the odds are that the problem will be a fairly short-lived mechanical one – sometimes known as 'plain, ordinary' back pain.

However, a minority of attacks of back pain are due to disc problems. And a far smaller minority are due to more serious causes.

So, in the next chapter, we'll look at what to do when 'plain, ordinary' back pain hits you.

4

What to do when you get an attack of backache

So what should you do when you get a pain in your back?

First, don't worry too much about what the actual diagnosis is. As we've seen in the last chapter, diagnosing backache is a very tricky business. And you're unlikely to be able to diagnose yourself.

However, do bear in mind that the odds are heavily in favour of the cause of the pain being something minor and transient. So you almost certainly *will* get better, provided you look after yourself and follow the guidelines in this chapter. We're going to be looking at simple things you can do in order to ease your pain and to speed recovery.

Should you see your doctor immediately?

But first, ought you to try and consult a doctor at once? No: bearing in mind that the pain might be gone by tomorrow, there's really not much point in tearing down to your GP's surgery. Nor is there anything to be gained by going off to A&E – where, to be frank, they are unlikely to be very enthusiastic about agreeing to see someone with backache.

Should you ask your doctor to come and see you? No. In any case, these days, it is becoming unlikely that you would succeed in getting a GP to make a 'house call' for a case of backache – unless you happen to have some other, more alarming symptoms.

However, if your back pain is bad, there is no harm in ringing your doctor's practice for advice, perhaps from the practice nurse. Some general practices will actually put you through to a 'duty doctor', although I'm afraid that is uncommon these days.

In the UK, an alternative is to ring NHS Direct (see Useful addresses at the back of this book). This is a government-backed answering scheme, staffed by very experienced nurses, and they can give you good general advice about your backache – advice that may well be along the lines of the guidelines in this chapter.

Another very valuable source of advice is slowly being introduced in the UK. In fact, it is already up and running in Scotland. It might well be termed 'Dial-a-Physio', because that is what it is!

The new scheme allows you to ring up an NHS physiotherapist directly, instead of having to go through the roundabout process of being referred by a GP. Physiotherapists are highly trained, and they know all about 'Red Flag' symptoms that might suggest that there is actually something serious wrong with you. As I have said before, that is rare. (Serious causes of back pain are dealt with in Chapter 12.)

When this scheme reaches your area, the idea is that on the phone the physiotherapist will ask you for details about your back pain. On the basis of what you tell her, she may:

- give you advice there and then;
- invite you to go to her clinic/department;
- suggest that it's time to see your GP.

Whether you've tried to get telephone advice or not, there may well come a time when your pain doesn't seem to be easing, and you decide to *try* to make an appointment to see your GP.

But please be aware that at present many UK general practices are running a bizarre scheme in which everybody who wants an appointment has to ring up at eight o'clock in the morning. Within 20 minutes or so, all the appointment 'slots' for the day have gone. This extraordinary system is operated so that practices can meet government targets for giving people 'same day appointments' – and so claim a financial reward ...

If your general practice is operating a 'patient-unfriendly' system like this, there is something to be said for switching to another one.

While you are waiting for an appointment with your GP, I suggest that you make sure that you try the simple measures for back pain outlined later in this chapter. What you can expect from your doctor, when you get to see her, is described in Chapter 5.

Should you immediately ring an osteopath or chiropractor?

Again, on the first day of your backache there's probably not much point in phoning to try to get an appointment with a 'manipulator', since you may well be OK by the next morning. But it might be worth ringing for simple advice – because some osteopaths and chiropractors are willing to give you helpful tips over the phone.

However, one thing to remember is that good manipulative practitioners are usually very heavily booked up for some days ahead. So there is something to be said for making an appointment – which you could always cancel later if you get better. Incidentally, unlike many general practices, chiropractors and osteopaths do *not* operate a 'you must ring at 8 a.m.' policy!

How can you find one to contact? There are three simple ways:

1 By telephone. To get the name of a qualified osteopath in your area, ring the General Osteopathic Council (see Useful addresses at the back of this book). To get the name of a chiropractor, ring the General Chiropractic Council. (Again, see Useful addresses.)
2 Via the internet (see General Osteopathic Council and General Chiropractic Council in Useful addresses. These give websites for registered osteopaths and qualified chiropractors.)
3 Through *Yellow Pages*. Look under 'Osteopaths' and you will find a large 'box' in which all the registered practitioners of your region are listed. The situation with chiropractors is slightly more complicated, as they are divided into different groups. But in most areas of the UK, if you look up 'Chiropractors' in *Yellow Pages* you will find a fairly big box listing all the members of the British Chiropractic Association (see Useful addresses).

It may well be that you will also find a smaller box in *Yellow Pages* placed by the McTimoney Chiropractic Association (see Useful addresses). This is a splinter group of chiropractors, but they too are registered with the General Chiropractic Council.

In South Welsh phone directories, there is also the relatively new Welsh Institute of Chiropractic, which is located near Pontypridd (again, details in Useful addresses).

There is a lot more information about osteopaths and chiropractors in Chapters 6 and 7.

Should you ring an unregistered manipulator?

Basically, no. Until the very late twentieth century, it was legal for *anyone* to put up a sign describing himself as 'an osteopath' or 'a chiropractor'. Indeed, in the 1970s I actually consulted an unqualified manipulator myself, mistakenly thinking that she was a fully trained osteopath – because that's what the notice-board in her front garden said. It was an interesting experience ...

I'm glad to say that the law has been tightened up a lot in recent years, and people are no longer allowed to pretend to be qualified in osteopathy or chiropractic. However, there are quite a few manipulators around who are *not* registered chiropractors or osteopaths. Some describe themselves – rather oddly – as 'physiologists'. Others call

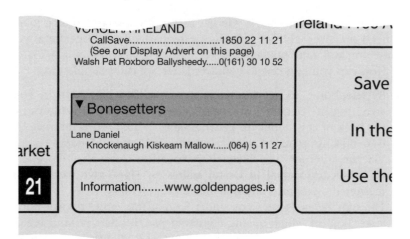

Figure 4.1 Bonesetter's listing in the Irish telephone directory

themselves 'sports manipulators'. For all I know, they may well be sincere, and they might do some good ... or not. My advice is to stick to a qualified osteopath or chiropractor.

What about bonesetters? This profession has a long, and mostly honourable, tradition, going back hundreds of years. But these manipulators have now all but disappeared from Britain.

However, on a recent visit to southern Ireland I discovered that the Irish *Golden Pages* still have a category headed 'Bonesetters' (see Figure 4.1). At least one such healer is at work in County Cork, and I hope to interview him about bonesetting on my next trip to the Emerald Isle.

Simple, self-help things you can do for your backache

Now let's look at straightforward, common-sense things that you can do for yourself when backache suddenly hits you.

First, *stop what you're doing.*

Why? Because there's a considerable chance that what you're doing when you first notice the pain is a contributory factor in causing your backache.

Are you mowing the lawn? Well, stop.

Are you carrying shopping bags? Well, put them down.

Are you playing golf? Then abandon the round, and walk off the course.

Are you sitting in a chair? Get out of it – because the shape of it may be bad for your back.

Are you stripping the bed? Then give up – and let somebody else do it.

Are you lifting heavy objects at work? Well, stop – and tell your boss that you can't lift any more today.

OK, I know that you're probably starting to say 'But …' However, I ask you to 'But me no buts'! You've got backache, and you need to take care of yourself.

In most people there's a rather endearing tendency to want to 'struggle on' and 'just finish this job' (or 'finish this game'). But don't do it. *Look after your back instead.*

Your best move now is to sit on a comfortable chair, or lie on a bed or couch. If possible, stay there for 20 or 30 minutes. Give your poor old back a chance to recover.

Keeping yourself warm and reducing pain

Nobody really knows why, but in general an attack of back pain will feel worse if you're cold. It's probably connected with the effect that coldness has on blood vessels, which is to make them get narrower.

Anyway, in the first couple of hours after you develop a backache, try to keep yourself not only comfortable, but reasonably warm. If you're at home, then the best thing of all would be to relax on your bed, and cover yourself with a cosy eiderdown or duvet. A lot of people get great relief from placing a hot water bottle – wrapped in a towel, to avoid burning – over the aching area of the back. In addition, warm 'wraps' – sold in pharmacies – have become very popular since early 2009.

Also, I suggest that you take a pain-killer as soon as possible. Aspirin, ibuprofen or paracetamol are all fine, provided that you haven't had any bad experiences with them in the past. However, the first two should *not* be taken on an empty stomach. (There's a lot more about pain-killers in Chapter 5.)

Use this couple of hours of rest, warmth and pain relief to relax as much as possible, and to see if your backache is getting better or not. If it *isn't*, then you must set about planning what you're going to do over the next few days. For instance:

- You may have to 'phone in sick' to your workplace.
- You may have to get someone to do things around the house for you.
- You may have to find someone to pick up the children from school.

- You may have to ring up and cancel any sporting arrangements you've got fixed (be firm!).
- You can try to decide whether you need any medical/osteopathic/ chiropractic help.

By the end of the first day, you need to have formulated a plan for what you're going to do if the pain persists for the next week or so. And if it does persist, then the rest of this chapter will help you to cope with it, by means of various 'self-help' methods.

If the pain continues …

So let's assume that the pain *didn't* go away on day one, and is clearly going to continue for a while. By now, you may have seen a doctor, osteopath or chiropractor, or are waiting to see one. But what can you do to help yourself?

Well, there are quite a few good self-help techniques. But perhaps the most important thing is *not* to do anything that could make your backache worse. In particular, avoid all bending and lifting.

I often give people that advice, and they usually nod their heads and say something like 'Certainly, doctor'. Then, if I don't stop them, they immediately bend over – and pick up some heavy briefcase or rucksack, or two-year-old, from the floor!

So take care of your back. You are currently 'walking wounded', and you really need to look after yourself until you're completely better.

Cold packs

Despite the fact that warmth usually alleviates pain, it's also true that putting a 'cold pack' on an area of backache will often give some relief. You can buy cold packs from any large pharmacy. The idea is that you put them in your fridge till they're really chilled, and then apply them to the area of pain for 15 or 20 minutes. *Take great care to wrap the pack in something like a towel, in order to protect your skin.*

If you don't want to go to the expense or trouble of buying a cold pack, then many people make do with a packet of frozen peas.

Exercise

You definitely should go in for some gentle exercise when you have a bad back. The worst possible thing you can do is to remain totally immobile, because that just makes everything stiffen up.

So what should you do in the way of exercise? If the weather is bad and you can't go out, try doing a little gentle dancing on the spot, plus waving your arms around to music. Don't be embarrassed about doing this! Working out to an aerobics DVD is OK, *provided* that you don't do any bending.

Gentle walking is generally good. So too is swimming – though it's better to splash about in the water rather than attempt anything too intensive. However, please note that the breaststroke puts quite a lot of strain on the upper part of the spine, and is best avoided when you have backache.

Although I certainly wouldn't recommend competitive sport for everyone, I find that – for me personally – gentle tennis is good when I have a backache. The action of stretching upwards to serve has often eased my discomfort considerably.

In general, golf is *not* good for backache – because of the classic rotatory motion of the swing, which twists the spine right round. So it may be sensible to stay off the links till you're better.

Working out gently in the gym under supervision is often helpful, but don't do it if it causes you pain.

This could be a good time to start developing your 'core strength' through exercise – see Chapter 13.

Stretching your spine

In most types of backache, it's usually a good idea to try stretching your spine. This can ease the pressure on complaining joints and muscles.

What you do is rather like an Alexander technique exercise (see Chapter 11). Stand up straight, with your hands by your sides. Now imagine that there's a little pulley attached to the top of your skull. Allow it to draw your head further and further upwards. If you do this properly, you will actually get half an inch or so taller. Hold the stretch for a minute or so, then relax. Repeat 10 times.

Another way of stretching your spine is advocated by some doctors, who tell those consulting them: 'Go and hang from the top of a door by your hands.' Frankly, I'm not too keen on the idea of dangling from a door! First, it hurts your hands a lot, unless you wear really thick gloves. Second, there is always the slight possibility that the door might suddenly come off its hinges …

An alternative that I've often used successfully is to go to your stairs, and hang a loop of stout rope across them from a couple of banister posts. (*Warning*: You must be absolutely sure that everything is secure, and that nothing could possibly give way under your weight.) Then

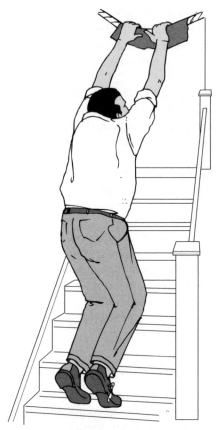

Figure 4.2 Stretching your spine on the stairs

stand on the stairs with your arms above your head, so that your hands can just grasp the rope. (If it's uncomfortable on your fingers, wrap the rope in a cloth.) See Figure 4.2.

Now gently take your feet an inch or two off the ground, so that your weight is entirely supported by your hands. The effect of this is to stretch most of your spine. I would recommend doing this 'stretch' for 10 seconds, then relaxing – and repeating 10 times.

In the unlikely event that this stretch causes you any pain, stop and consult your doctor, physiotherapist, osteopath or chiropractor.

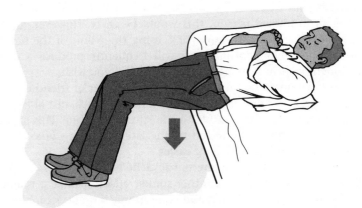

Figure 4.3 'Delvin's lumbar stretch manoeuvre' for pain in the lower back

The lumbar stretch manoeuvre

This is for lumbar (i.e. low) backache. Many years ago, when I was getting a lot of back pain in the lower back, I came up with this simple technique for stretching the lumbar spine. I described it in the magazine *World Medicine*, and a number of doctors wrote to me to say that they too had found it helpful.

What you do is shown in Figure 4.3. Lie on a firm bed or divan with your feet on the ground. Shunt your body gently forward in the direction of your legs, until your bottom is just off the edge. The rest of your trunk – that is, from about the waist up – is still on the bed.

Now let your bottom drop downwards as much as you can, while still keeping the top half of you on the divan. This stretches out your lumbar spine a few centimetres. Keep your bottom in this 'dropped' position for about five minutes. With luck, at the end of that time you will feel a slight easing of the pain.

Massage from your partner

Surprisingly, gentle massage from a partner or friend can often ease backache. This may well be because it relieves the tension in over-stretched muscles.

Begin by stripping down to your underwear. Then lie flat on your face on the bed. The other person – who *must* have warm hands – should sit down beside you, facing towards your head.

Don't get your friend or partner to attempt any kind of manipulation. For an untrained person, this would be crazy. However, gentle rubbing movements on the bare back, using the palms of the hands, can be astonishingly soothing and will frequently produce a rapid improvement in pain levels. Use a massage oil if you wish.

Another extremely useful thing that your partner or friend can try is to gently press the tips of the thumbs into your back, just alongside the spine and as near as possible to the site of the pain. This simple technique – which was pioneered by the late Dr James Cyriax – will very often make things quite a lot easier.

Some people who have long-term backache buy themselves a 'spine prodder' – a device that has a rather similar effect. It's like a walking stick with two sharp bends in it, and you can buy it quite cheaply from shops specializing in back pain. It works best on pain in the thoracic (i.e. chest) region of your spine.

Gentle traction from a partner

A few couples who have long experience of back pain have discovered for themselves the fact that it often helps if one partner stretches the other's spine by gently pulling the legs downwards, or the arms upwards, while the person with backache is lying on a bed. But stop if it causes any pain at all.

It is really best if you get a physiotherapist or other health professional to show you how to do this. (*Most important*: The partner who is doing the soothing traction should take great care not to put his/her own back out. Don't pull hard – and stop if you feel any discomfort yourself.)

Sorting out your bed

Speaking of beds, anyone who has just developed backache should think about whether the thing we spend eight hours a night on could be partly responsible. Yes, I'm talking about your bed.

From my years of doing home visits in general practice, I would say that a small proportion of people sleep on beds that are very old and have collapsed in some way. Sometimes, the mattress has split down the middle, and they haven't noticed it. That's particularly common in older folk who haven't bought a new bed or mattress in 40 years.

Sleeping on something that is totally 'clapped out' is really not good for your spine, because it lets it sag badly in the middle of the night. You may even find that you wake up every morning with a pain – which gradually goes off during the day.

Now, I don't want to over-emphasize the role of beds and mattresses in back pain. To be frank, the bed-manufacturing industry does tend to exaggerate the problems that bedding can cause. Naturally, they want to sell you new beds – and so they stress the fact that buying a nice replacement might help your spine.

I feel you should be a little cautious in accepting these arguments. Be particularly wary of firms that want to sell you 'orthopaedic beds' or 'orthopaedic mattresses'. In this context, the word 'orthopaedic' is practically meaningless. Unfortunately, any manufacturer can call his product 'orthopaedic'.

If you like the feel of a particular bed or mattress, and are comfortable after lying on it for half an hour in the shop, then fair enough. But don't imagine that an orthopaedic surgeon has decided that it will cure your backache. It probably won't.

So if you fancy changing your bed, in the hope that this will improve your back symptoms, what should you do?

I think you should go to a reputable bedding shop and try lying on the beds – preferably with your partner – for a good long time. Don't let yourself be rushed.

As you might guess, I would recommend that you look for a bed with a firm mattress. Indeed, during a survey on beds that I did for a national newspaper I discovered that these days virtually *all* customers ask for a firm mattress. It's a little difficult to imagine anyone asking for one that *wasn't* firm. However, you don't need to get yourself a bed that feels as hard as concrete; some 'give' in it is essential, to accommodate the natural curves of your body.

One final point: make sure that when they deliver the bed, the company will actually *assemble* it for you. I've encountered one or two firms that – astonishingly enough – expected you to put your own bed together. This is not a great idea when you already have a bad back.

Summing up

So it's clear that there are various useful things you can do to help yourself in the first few days after getting backache.

The best ones are gentle exercise, cold packs, massage and stretching exercises – and, above all, treating your back carefully and avoiding lifting.

However, if your back pain is bad, you obviously *have* to put yourself in the hands of the professionals. And, in the next four chapters, I'll explain what they can do to help you.

5

Getting help from a doctor

If you're lucky, your backache may go away after a few days, particularly if you've been using common-sense self-help measures, like avoiding lifting and bending. (A lot of these self-help strategies are described in Chapter 4.)

But what if it *won't* go away? In this case, you're going to need professional assistance. In the UK and most other Western countries, the professions that can provide skilled help for your back are these:

- doctors;
- osteopaths;
- chiropractors;
- physiotherapists.

This chapter – and the three that follow it – will tell you about these four types of professional, and what they can do to help you.

Symptoms that mean you need professional help

First of all, let's look at symptoms that mean you really should seek medical help. In my view, these are the ones that mean 'see an expert':

- backache that has gone on for more than a week;
- backache that is really agonizing – the kind that makes you cry out with pain;
- backache that is obviously going to make it impossible for you to do your job for some time;
- backache that makes it difficult for you to walk;
- backache associated with pain down your legs or arms.

In addition, there are certain things that are described as 'Red Flag' symptoms – because they could indicate something serious. They include:

- back pain after a bad accident;
- back pain that is associated with difficulty in passing urine;

- back pain associated with lack of control of the bowels;
- back pain with numbness around the genitals or the anus, or the area in between;
- back pain with disturbance of sexual function;
- back pain with any kind of paralysis;
- back pain in a person who has had cancer;
- back pain in a person who is taking steroids;
- back pain in someone who has HIV;
- back pain with marked weight loss;
- back pain happening at the same time as a severe generalized illness.

In addition, there are two 'age-related' factors that indicate you should see a doctor. They are:

- If you're under 25 and male, and keep getting bad pain in your lower back, you should consult your GP – this is because there is a risk that you might have ankylosing spondylitis (see Chapter 12).
- If you're over 60 when persistent pain first occurs, you should check with your GP because of the small risk of cancer – however, please remember that it's much more likely that you just have 'rheumatism' or osteoarthritis. (A degree of osteoarthritis can be found in almost everybody's spines after the age of 60.)

Now we'll look at what doctors can do for your backache.

Getting help from a family doctor

In most instances, this means getting help from your GP – although later in this chapter we'll also deal with other, more specialized, types of doctor.

In the UK, almost everybody is registered with a GP. The same isn't true in all parts of Europe, but in Ireland, France, Spain and most EU countries there are family doctors or generalists who are a good 'first port of call' when you run into trouble with your back.

In some Commonwealth countries, that is no longer the case. Indeed, I am told that in Australia people who have backache are now more likely to find an osteopath than to seek out a doctor.

Nevertheless, in the UK it's mainly to GPs that those with back pain turn initially. And, in theory, your general practitioner should be reasonably good at managing backache. After all, she sees roughly a dozen cases of it per week.

I have to admit that when speaking privately, chiropractors and osteopaths often criticize GPs, saying that they 'don't really know very much about backache', and that all they do is 'dish out pills and certificates'. Sadly, in some poor-quality surgeries – particularly in inner cities – that may well be the case. I have to admit there are still some pretty awful doctors, though they are much fewer and farther between than they used to be. This is mainly because GPs now have to submit to regular assessments of their skills and of their ability to keep up to date with modern medicine.

Unfortunately, it remains true that most doctors were taught virtually nothing about backache at medical school. Generally speaking, their professors and lecturers were busy teaching rather more glamorous subjects, like cardiology and transplant surgery. So the majority of GPs have had to acquire their knowledge of back pain as best they can.

However, let's assume that you have a good and well-informed family doctor. What can she do for you when you go to see her?

Well, first of all please bear in mind that when you walk into her consulting room you have a 'slot' of 10 minutes. (There are still a few dreadful practices where people are only 'allowed' *five* minutes.) This 10-minute period is quite a contrast with the half-hour to an hour that you will get at an osteopath's or chiropractor's.

So it's clearly important that you utilize your 10 minutes to the best advantage. Before you go in, be prepared, so you are ready to tell the doctor your story clearly. Don't waste your time by ambling in slowly, admiring the view outside her surgery window, and then saying vague things like 'I don't really know where to begin ...' Instead, just tell her that you've got a pain in your back, and the length of time you have had it.

Questions that she should ask you include:

- Whereabouts in your back is the pain?
- When did you first notice it?
- What were you doing at the time?
- In the day or two beforehand, had you done anything out of the ordinary (like lifting furniture, or trying ten-pin bowling)?
- Does anything make it worse – like standing up, lifting, sneezing or coughing?
- Most importantly, does the pain run down the back or side of your leg?

Why is this last question so vital? Because pain that runs from the lower part of the spine and down your leg, in the general direction of your heel, is very likely to be caused by pressure on a nerve root in the lumbar area. And that is most often caused by a bulging ('slipped') disc.

A disc problem is of much more significance than most other types of back pain, because it is likely to go on for quite a long time. Also, it may need surgery in order to correct it. Disc-induced pain is dealt with in Chapter 10. Happily, most cases of backache are *not* caused by disc trouble.

Nurse practitioner

Although most consultations in general practice are with GPs, these days you may sometimes find yourself seeing a 'nurse practitioner' instead.

These are very highly trained nurses who are taking on an increasing amount of the family doctor's workload. They do a very good job. However, it is obvious that there has to be a limit as to what they know about the spine and its disorders. So there may perhaps be times when you would prefer to specify that you want to see a doctor instead. This should not offend anyone.

Medical examination

Now the doctor needs to examine you. A good tip is to be prepared for this by arriving in clothes that are easily removed. Wearing eight layers of togs that need to be taken off one at a time is not a good plan, because it will mean that a large chunk of your slot is wasted in dressing and undressing.

Most GPs don't need you to undress completely, but ideally a man should strip down to his underpants, and a woman to her bra and pants. Some people are reluctant to agree to this disrobing, and say things like 'But there's nothing to see, doc'.

However, the point is that a good doctor needs to look at the whole length of your spine, and see if there are any unusual curves or other abnormalities. She can also assess whether the muscles are in spasm around your area of pain. She can observe what your posture is like, and whether you are standing with one shoulder higher than the other.

What else happens? Different medics have different ideas about how to examine a back, but a common scheme is this:

1 The doctor asks you to stand as straight as you can, with both heels together, and inspects your entire back.
2 She asks you to bend forward, as if trying to touch your toes; this enables her to assess the forward flexibility of your spine.

3 She asks you to bend *backwards* – supporting you from behind if you feel unsteady; this gives her a good assessment of the rearward flexibility of the spine.

4 She then gets you to run your hand down your right leg, as far as you can; this lets her assess lateral flexion.

5 Next, she asks you to run your hand down the outside of the left leg; this gives an assessment of lateral flexibility in the other direction.

6 Following this, she presses your spine and adjoining areas, using her fingertips or thumbs, trying to find a point of maximum tenderness; very often, this gives accurate information about precisely where the seat of the trouble is.

7 Experienced doctors will also try pressing on your two sacro-iliac joints to see if they are tender. As explained in Chapter 2, the S-I joint is located near the top of the buttock – and is a more common cause of pain than is generally realized.

8 Very often, your doctor will now get you to lie on your back on the couch, with your knees straight. She will then *lift* your legs, one after the other. The degree to which she can lift your leg upwards without causing you pain is important, because if it is less than normal, that will often indicate possible disc trouble. This examination is called 'Straight Leg Raising', and the doctor will usually record the result in your notes, using an abbreviation such as 'SLR 90 degrees' or 'SLR zero degrees'. A figure of 90 degrees is very good, and zero degrees is bad – because it suggests that a disc may be pressing on nerve roots.

If she has any suspicion that you might have a nerve root compression – for instance, caused by a bulging disc – she should go on to do a brief neurological (nervous system) examination, to see if the nerves in your legs are affected. That would mean testing your reflexes with a little hammer, and checking whether you have lost any sensation in the lower part of your legs.

So, at the end of all that, a skilled doctor will have a reasonable idea of what sort of shape you're in. But, as I explained in Chapter 3, it's unlikely that she will be able to give you a precise diagnosis. She should, though, certainly be able to tell you whether there is any sign of disc trouble, or whether the problem seems to be a milder mechanical one.

As I've said repeatedly, most cases of backache *are* due to minor mechanical difficulties, and can be expected to improve soon if treated with care. Many such pains will be completely gone within a few weeks – if they are not aggravated any further by, say, heavy lifting.

Note: These days, your GP is very unlikely to order an X-ray of your back. This is because X-rays aren't usually of any help, and also they subject you to a small dose of radiation. Also, hospital Radiology Departments now tend to refuse to do them in cases of backache.

Treatment from your GP

So what will your GP do for you? Let me stress that she is most unlikely to attempt any manipulation of your spine. This is in sharp contrast to the approach of osteopaths and chiropractors. The vast majority of doctors have not been trained in manipulation; and, even if they had the time to do it, they wouldn't know how.

A very tiny number of doctors have been trained in manipulation by the London College of Osteopathic Medicine, which currently graduates about five medics each year. So it is most unlikely that your GP will have studied there.

This is not your doctor's fault. It's just the way things are. Your GP will, however, give you good advice about looking after yourself and relieving your pain. In summary, this advice is likely to be along these lines:

- Don't lift anything (except teacups and other light objects) till you're better.
- Keep yourself warm.
- Rest – this doesn't mean that you should go and lie immobile on a hard board for six weeks; it means 'take things easy'.
- Avoid any sport that might make things worse (alas, that's most of them).
- If you're doing a 'heavy' job – like brick-laying or plumbing – stay off work for a while (admittedly, that's very difficult for many people these days).

This brings us to the question of the dreaded 'certificate'. Getting a National Insurance medical certificate – or 'a doctor's line' or 'a doctor's paper', as it's known in some parts of the UK – is a major reason why so many people still go to their GPs with backache.

You see, osteopaths, chiropractors and physiotherapists cannot issue these much-prized little slips of paper. They can write you a *private* certificate, to keep your boss happy. But to all intents and purposes, National Insurance certificates for back pain are only signed by GPs.

Some years ago, the authorities did something quite sensible in ruling that people could 'self-certificate' – that is, fill in their own National Insurance certificate – for illnesses of up to seven days' duration. But if you're off work for longer than that, you will need an official form signed by a doctor. (*Note*: This system is due to change substantially in 2009 or 2010.)

If you need a 'doctor's certificate', don't forget to ask your GP for one while you're in her surgery. Otherwise, you can waste quite a bit of time and effort trying to get one later. Please note that a doctor cannot sign a certificate for back pain or anything else unless she has actually *seen* you. Some people still ring their GP's surgery and say 'Oh, I've got backache; could the doc just leave a certificate out for me?' To do that would be illegal.

Drugs prescribed by GPs

Now, what about medication? If you go and see a doctor because you've got backache, there's a very high chance that she will offer you a prescription for a drug. If you are already treating yourself with something, please tell her – because (a) she may have been about to give you the same thing; (b) what she prescribes might clash with what you're already taking.

So what medications could your GP prescribe you for your back?

Well, can I begin by stressing that there isn't a drug known to science that can actually *cure* a back problem. People find this hard to believe, and think that there must be pills that will somehow put everything right. This is not the case. No drug can make a bulging disc go back, or persuade a subluxated facet joint to leap back into place.

But faith in pills can be a very important thing. Many years ago, there was a medication called 'Lobak'. The name was brilliant, because it suggested that the pill would go straight to the person's lower back, and make it all better. The product was very cleverly marketed to doctors – some of whom seemed to swallow the advertising claims wholeheartedly – and many members of the public also got to know about it.

The result was that hundreds of thousands of people were prescribed Lobak. They told their friends about it, and their pals went along to *their* doctors and also asked for it. If you were put on Lobak, you really felt that something was being done for your lower spine.

The reality, of course, was that Lobak was simply an effective but minor pain-killer. It didn't target the lower back – or anywhere else – at all. After many years of fame, it became less fashionable, and it was eventually withdrawn. It is possible that one factor in its eclipse was the gradual realization that 'Lobak' is also the name of a sort of Malaysian pork sausage, braised in soy sauce!

So if drugs can't actually cure your backache, what can they do?

The medications that your GP is likely to prescribe for you may do two things:

- relieve your pain;
- reduce inflammation.

What is the point of reducing inflammation? Well, it is thought that in many cases of back pain, inflammation develops around the original lesion.

In practice, a lot of the products that GPs prescribe for backache are pain-relieving *and* anti-inflammatory. In other words, they do both jobs.

Until recently, it was also quite common for those with back pain to be put on 'muscle relaxants'. That has become rarer these days, partly because it is doubtful if these products did much good. Also, some of them were actually tranquillizers and we now know that practically all tranquillizers can have serious side-effects – especially the risk of you becoming addicted to them.

So which back-pain pills should you be on? Some people would say, 'Oh that's entirely up to the doc, isn't it?' But these days, people have an increasing say in what is prescribed for them, and sensible doctors are willing to go along with that.

For instance, you may well be aware that a certain drug (or group of drugs) has upset you in the past. Or you may know that you get on particularly well with a certain product. In both cases, please do tell the doctor, before she writes her prescription. It's your body, and you are entitled to have some input into the choice of medication.

So, what drugs are available for backache these days?

Paracetamol

I should stress at the outset that ordinary paracetamol (also known as 'acetaminophen' in many parts of the world) is quite often as effective as anything in relieving pain and reducing inflammation. People tend not to 'rate' paracetamol, because of the fact that you can buy it over the counter (OTC), as well as on a doctor's prescription.

In reality, it is a good and safe drug, as long as you do not exceed the maximum dose, which is 4 g (that is, eight 500 mg tablets) per day. Experts particularly recommend it for *elderly* people with backache, because it is free of some of the dangerous side-effects that other drugs often cause in older folk.

However, like any other medication, paracetamol can have ill-effects. These are rare, but they include rashes and blood problems.

Generally speaking, the drug should not be used by people who have liver damage or kidney disease, or who are dependent on alcohol.

Paracetamol is contained in many, many preparations, including well-known ones like Panadol, Anadin Extra and Disprol. It's important for you to realize this, because if your GP prescribes you a paracetamol-containing medication for your backache, you should *not* take a paracetamol-containing OTC product as well. This would probably result in an overdose.

Aspirin

What about aspirin? Again, people tend to think that aspirin is just a 'trivial' drug, but in fact it's a jolly good medication for backache – so don't be surprised if your GP prescribes an aspirin-containing product for you.

However, aspirin is fairly notorious for sometimes causing side-effects, particularly in elderly people. The chief one is irritation of the stomach's lining – which may progress to internal bleeding. This can be very serious indeed.

So if your doctor prescribes you an aspirin-containing medication, make sure that you don't take it on an empty stomach. The pharmacist should advise you to take it 'after meals', which should protect your gastric lining. But if it seems to be causing you pain in your abdomen, stop taking it, and let your GP know.

Other, less common, side-effects of aspirin include asthma, skin reactions and ringing in the ears. If you develop any of them, cease taking the aspirin.

And if your GP prescribes aspirin for your back, please *don't* also take one of the dozens of aspirin-containing medications that are available as OTC products from pharmacies, supermarkets, shops and petrol stations. These include Aspro, Disprin and Anadin.

Non-steroidal anti-inflammatory drugs

At the moment, the medications that GPs are most likely to prescribe for backache are the group called 'non-steroidal anti-inflammatory drugs'. This cumbersome title is usually abbreviated to 'NSAIDs' – often pronounced 'enn-sayds'. You probably know the names of several NSAIDs, because so many people use them. Currently, the best-known one in the UK is ibuprofen, also marketed as Nurofen, Fenbid and Brufen.

NSAIDs work in much the same way as aspirin does, and some doctors think that they are really not much better than aspirin. But they do have good pain-relieving qualities, as well as the ability to reduce inflammation.

Their various manufacturers make extravagant claims about whether one or other of them is superior to the rest, but in fact they are all about as powerful as each other.

However, there is a lot of variation in how those with back pain react to them. Roughly 60 per cent of people respond well to *any* NSAID, but the other 40 per cent of the population will do better on one NSAID rather than another. Unfortunately, you can only find out which NSAID is best for you by trial and error. What this means is that if one brand of pills doesn't seem to be working very well on your back, you should ask your doctor about switching you to another one.

Well-known and long-established NSAIDs used for back pain include:

- diclofenac (Voltarol);
- ibuprofen (Brufen, Fenbid, Nurofen);
- fenbufen (Lederfen);
- fenoprofen (Fenopron);
- indometacin (Indocid);
- ketoprofen (Orudis);
- mefenamic acid (Ponstan);
- meloxicam (Mobic);
- naproxen (Naprosyn);
- suldinac (Clinoril);
- tenoxicam (Mobiflex);
- tiaprofenic acid (Surgam).

It is vitally important for those with backache to realize that NSAID medications can have significant side-effects. These include:

- abdominal pain;
- nausea;
- diarrhoea;
- and sometimes, bleeding from the stomach.

There are many other possible side-effects of NSAIDs (including skin rashes, asthma attacks and dizziness), but it is gastric bleeding that is most likely to lead to life-threatening illness. So please take your NSAID precisely as prescribed, and do not be tempted to exceed the stated dose – even when your back pain is bad.

Often, when GPs prescribe NSAIDs for those with back pain, they will try to prevent gastric problems by also giving a supply of 'stomach-protective' drugs called 'proton-pump inhibitors'. The best known of these is omeprazole (also known as Losec).

If you get any symptoms that indicate you might have bleeding in the stomach, please stop taking the pills at once, and seek medical help. Symptoms of bleeding from the stomach lining include:

- vomiting blood or, more usually, what looks like 'coffee-ground' material;
- passing black, tarry motions;
- abdominal pain.

At the beginning of the twenty-first century, there was much fanfare about an entirely new class of NSAIDs, which were supposed to be much safer for those with back pain (and others) to take. They are called 'the Cox-2 inhibitors'. Alas, these 'wonder drugs' turned out to sometimes cause thrombotic (i.e. clotting) problems, including heart attacks and strokes.

Things then got worse. In the last few years, it's become clear that even the 'traditional' NSAIDs may be associated with a small increased risk of thrombosis – particularly when used for a long period of time, and at high dosage.

I don't think you need to get excessively worried about all this, if your GP just prescribes you a modest dose of an NSAID for a short period of time. If it's any reassurance, when I have a bit of backache, I quite often take one myself.

However, it is *not* a good idea for people with back pain to go on and on swallowing NSAIDs for months on end, unless there is some very compelling medical reason for having such a prolonged course.

Note: Some NSAIDs can be taken in suppository form.

Warning: If you have an active peptic ulcer (gastric or duodenal) you should not be taking an NSAID – no matter how bad your back pain is.

Straightforward pain-killers

As an alternative to NSAIDs, your GP may prescribe straightforward pain-killers (analgesics). There are dozens of these, but a lot of them contain codeine, the well-known anti-pain drug.

Codeine is chemically related to morphine and pethidine, but is much milder. It has no anti-inflammatory effect, but it does relieve back pain very well. It is also remarkably free of side-effects much of the time, except that most people who take it are likely to become rather constipated.

Usually, they are not too bothered about this, as long as their backache is being eased. However, it isn't a good idea to keep on taking codeine for a long time, because your bowels are likely to become rather sluggish.

There is an extraordinary number of 'combination products' that combine codeine with other things – particularly paracetamol. Doctors prescribe these 'mix and match' medications quite a bit for backache, though experts tend to be a little doubtful about whether there is much point in such combinations.

Extremely strong analgesics

There also exist certain *very* strong pain-killers, mostly of the 'opioid' group – which means related to opium. Your GP will only prescribe these if you are getting truly awful back pain.

In general, they should only be used for very short periods, because they have all sorts of side-effects – like nausea, vomiting, constipation and gall bladder problems. They can affect the mind, causing mood changes, drowsiness and hallucinations. (For this reason, they are widely sought after by drug addicts.) Very importantly, they are seriously habituating.

So if your doctor feels that your back pain merits a prescription for the strongest type of pain-killer, you should try to take it for the shortest time possible. Never exceed the prescribed dose. And do *not* drink alcohol while you are on it; the combination could knock you right out, and could just possibly be fatal.

Skin applications

Some GPs prescribe skin applications, which you rub into your back. These days, they very often contain NSAIDs (see p. 46). Common brands are:

- Ketoprofen Gel;
- Feldene Gel;
- Fenbid Forte Gel;
- Ibugel Forte;
- Oruvail Gel;
- Powergel;
- Traxam Foam;
- Voltarol Emulgel.

The general idea is that when you rub these gels or foams into your back, the NSAID will be absorbed deeply enough to relieve pain and ease inflammation. I have to be frank and say that some doctors are doubtful that any drug could achieve this degree of penetration through your skin and various other layers of tissue.

None the less, many of those with back pain do feel that they receive considerable benefit from these products. It is possible that the mere process of rubbing the gel/foam in – which is, after all, a form of massage – helps a lot.

There are also older non-NSAID products, of the type that sports coaches and masseurs have traditionally used. These include things like Tiger Balm and capsaicin cream (Zacin). They are thought to work by the principle of 'counter-irritation'; that is, they create a harmless irritation in your skin, so that it feels hot – and that makes the nearby pain more bearable.

In practice, if you have pain in your back it may sometimes be difficult to reach round and rub anything into the affected area. So you would probably need to have a partner or friend do the massaging in for you. If you can't do it yourself, and you don't have anyone who could help you, then there wouldn't be much point in accepting a prescription for one of the above-mentioned skin applications.

In summary, there are many medications that your GP can give you for backache. But, in general, they are things that will simply ease your pain while (I hope) your body gradually gets better. None of the above products is actually curative.

Getting help from other types of doctor

In the UK, the NHS system is such that you start by going to a GP – who may refer you to a more specialized doctor if necessary.

That is not the case in most other countries, where a lot of people choose to go directly to a specialist. In the UK, the only way of doing this would be to 'go privately'. Some people with back pain do this, completely bypassing their GPs.

To be honest, I don't really recommend taking that step. It would be very difficult for you, as a member of the public, to pick out precisely the type of specialist you need. You see, there are few doctors in the UK (or southern Ireland) who could accurately be described as 'back-pain specialists', and you won't find such a category in the *Yellow Pages* or the *Golden Pages*.

In reality, most of the consultants who you might go and see about your back pain would deal with a lot of other things as well. They are not treating backache all day and every day.

Nevertheless, there are types of specialist to whom your GP might well refer you if things get bad and if your back trouble is not clearing up. Here they are:

- Orthopaedic surgeons. The 'orthopods' are men (yes, I'm afraid they're still nearly always male!) who operate on bones, joints and muscles. A lot of their work is on the legs, arms and shoulders. Many of them do see people who have backache – and they end up operating on some of them (for instance, to remove a damaged disc).

- Neurosurgeons. These specialists are experts in problems of the nervous system, which includes the brain and the spinal cord. They tend to be very precise people, who are extremely good at detailed work with their hands. When I had my own disc operated on, I chose a neurosurgeon to do it.

- Rheumatologists. These are doctors who specialize in 'the rheumatic diseases', which means a wide variety of disorders of the joints and connective tissues. Some of them are very interested in back problems. Being doctors rather than surgeons, they do not operate.

- Orthopaedic doctors. There are not all that many of these. In the UK, the first of them was the late, great Dr James Cyriax of St Thomas' Hospital. Today, his methods are followed and developed by the Society of Orthopaedic Medicine and the Irish Society of Orthopaedic Medicine. Such specialists co-operate closely with physiotherapists, as Cyriax did. They lay great emphasis on very precise diagnosis of spinal and other problems, and treat them with such techniques as deep transverse friction (with the hands), manipulation and injection.

- Pain clinic specialists. In the UK and some other countries, there is now a good network of hospital clinics where specialists are devoted to relieving pain – from back trouble or any other cause. The consultants are often anaesthetists – because a lot of the practice of anaesthetics is about abolishing pain. They use techniques such as acupuncture and electro-stimulation as well as oral drugs and injections – and also psychotherapy. They are in the business of *relieving* your pain, rather than trying to cure the underlying cause. (For more information about pain clinics, see the website listed under Useful addresses at the end of this book.)

That's all I have to say about medical doctors. Let's move on now to the manipulators – and particularly to osteopaths and chiropractors.

6

Getting help from an osteopath

These days, huge numbers of people with back pain go to osteopaths, or to chiropractors. A lot of those consulting me ask: 'What's the *difference* between osteopathy and chiropractic?'

I'm inclined to reply 'Not very much' – though that reply will annoy many osteopaths and chiropractors! But as someone who has undergone a lot of treatment – much of it pretty successful – by practitioners from the two disciplines, I can say that being on the receiving end does frequently feel much the same in both cases.

Differences and similarities between osteopaths and chiropractors

Similarities

Both types of therapy rely largely on manipulating the spine and the nearby structures – though chiropractors refer to it as 'adjustment' rather than 'manipulation'.

Both disciplines were started by charismatic North Americans, in the late nineteenth century. And both of these founders had the idea that a lot of disease was caused by some sort of malposition of the spine.

Nevertheless, today many practitioners from both schools of thought seem to concentrate mainly on trying to use spinal adjustments to improve *backache* – rather than using it to try to cure, say, indigestion or constipation.

Differences

Osteopathy has traditionally employed quite a lot of 'leverage from a distance' in its manipulations, with short manual thrusts towards your spine. Chiropractic adjustments are generally more direct, working on the joints they want to affect, or the adjacent area.

Chiropractors quite often use X-rays. Osteopaths do not, and are very unlikely to have X-ray equipment on the premises.

In the UK, chiropractors refer to themselves as being 'chiropractic Doctors' – usually with a capital 'D', for some reason. Osteopaths rarely use the word 'doctor'.

Chiropractic clinics tend to market themselves quite enthusiastically, with large newspaper ads and even radio commercials. Osteopaths generally do not.

Er ... that's about it! Doubtless, I shall now receive letters from chiropractors and osteopaths who want to stress that their ways of working are very different. But, frankly, that has not been my experience as a person being treated.

History of osteopathy

Do please skip this bit if you are not very interested in history. However, the story of how osteopaths established themselves – against enormous opposition from the orthodox medical profession – is interesting. And it does help to explain the way in which they treat those with backache today.

Osteopathy was invented in about 1874 by Andrew Still (1828–1917), who was a qualified doctor, working in the American Mid-West. Orthodox medicine was pretty primitive at that time, and there was remarkably little that doctors could do for a lot of medical conditions – including backache.

Having lost several of his children to what was probably meningitis, Dr Still decided – not unreasonably – to try to establish a new system of medical treatment. He came to the conclusion that malalignment of the bones in the spine affected blood flow to the organs, and thus caused disease.

He seems to have developed a lot of skill in palpating (i.e. feeling) the spinal bones, and in manipulating them. He had clearly learned quite a lot from the old 'bone-setters', who knew that it was possible to move the vertebrae around, causing a satisfying and impressive 'click' – and sometimes relieving the person's pain. Indeed, he referred to himself as 'the lightning bone-setter'.

There were suggestions that Andrew Still could 'see under the skin' or had 'clairvoyant powers'. As you can imagine, all this did *not* go down a storm with the other members of the American medical profession! As a result, he branched away from orthodox medicine, and founded his own 'American School of Osteopathy' at Kirksville, Missouri, in 1892–3. His first graduate was a woman – which must have been quite a shock to some people at that time.

By the time Still died, during the First World War, osteopathy was thriving in great areas of the USA, but was constantly ridiculed by the American Medical Association who thought it dangerous and unscientific. Sometime in the twentieth century, the idea that 'the osteopathic lesion' somehow affected the blood supply to all the body's organs seems to have been quietly dropped by many osteopaths – but certainly not by all. Others believed – like chiropractors – that spinal adjustment could alter the *nerve* supply to various organs.

In the UK, the British Association of Osteopaths was formed in 1911. But for many decades, osteopathy was fiercely opposed by the UK medical profession, and particularly by the General Medical Council. A doctor who associated with an osteopath could be struck off – though I'm not sure that anyone ever really was.

During the years after the Second World War, the British public still had little idea of what osteopaths were. In 1963, the image of the profession was not greatly helped when the unfortunate 'society osteopath' Stephen Ward became a central figure in the national scandal that involved Christine Keeler and John Profumo.

In the 1970s, it was commonplace for members of the medical profession to mock osteopathy. As late as 1980, relations between doctors and osteopaths were so bad that I actually wrote a satirical weekly 'photo-story strip' in a medical newspaper, telling the tragic tale of a GP who had the misfortune to fall desperately in love with a beautiful osteopath. I think it was called 'Forbidden Passion ...'

In the UK, things began to change in the late 1980s when various bodies who represented osteopaths managed to resolve their differences and form a unified profession. In 1993, the Osteopathy Act was passed by Parliament. This set up the General Osteopathic Council, whose job is to regulate the profession, and ensure adequate training – generally leading to the award of a degree in about four years.

Since then, osteopathy has really gone from strength to strength in the UK. Its practitioners are respected, and the best ones have full books – and appreciable waiting lists for appointments. Most of the public have faith in what osteopathic treatment can do for people's 'bad backs'. There are now just over four thousand British osteopaths, and they treat about thirty thousand people every day. HRH Prince Charles is an enthusiastic supporter, and says he is proud of the fact that he played a small part in helping osteopathy to become a statutory profession.

Happily, many doctors have become far more open-minded about osteopathic practice, though there are still quite a few GPs who wouldn't dream of sending someone to an osteopath. Oddly, there is still some suspicion of osteopathy among certain religious groups. If you check the internet, you will find that there are articles that say things like: 'From a Christian perspective ... osteopathy is not a therapy to be recommended.' Apparently, the basis for this viewpoint is that Andrew Still was involved in 'psychic practices, particularly in his diagnostic methods'.

I cannot say that I have ever encountered any 'psychic practices' among the many osteopaths I have consulted – though there was one chap in Cambridge who used to go off and meditate briefly in a corner before manipulating my back. I didn't mind!

What happens when you consult an osteopath?

In Chapter 4, I explained how you can find a qualified osteopath. Nowadays, that's not difficult. In the UK, it is now (I am glad to say) illegal to *pretend* to be on the osteopathic register – so ideally you shouldn't encounter any 'bogus osteopaths'. However, in the last couple of years the courts have convicted 11 'practitioners' of falsely claiming to be trained osteopaths.

Having rung up for an appointment, you may well have to wait a few days, because osteopathic practitioners are now so popular. But when you finally get there, what happens?

Well, what takes place will vary a bit from practice to practice. But based on my own experience, I would say that all osteopaths begin by spending a fair amount of time taking a detailed 'history' of how you got your backache, how long you've had it, what makes it worse, what makes it better, and so on. They will also be interested in what you actually do in the course of your work, and while engaging in your hobbies and sports.

An osteopath might well allow 10 or 15 minutes trying to get an impression of you 'as a whole'. This is a big contrast with medicine in general practice, where your *entire* consultation with your GP is unlikely to last more than 10 minutes. Of course, in the case of an osteopathic consultation, a major factor is that *you* are paying. (More about fees in a moment.)

Next, the osteopath will examine you. For this, you really do need to overcome any modesty scruples you have, and remove most of your clothes. Men really need to strip down to their underpants, and women to their bra and pants. However, if you are really shy, some osteopaths will try to examine you through your clothes – or at least through a surgical gown.

The osteopath will probably do a physical examination like the one described in the previous chapter, with the object of assessing how flexible your spine is – bending forwards, backwards and sideways.

Also, while you are standing up he may well palpate your back (i.e. examine it with his fingers), to find out – among other things – how the bones are aligned, whether your muscles are in spasm, and where the tender spots are.

After that, the osteopath will ask you to get on his couch. These couches are generally nicely padded and a pleasure to relax on – with an aperture to breathe through while you are lying face down. But if you're not comfortable, just say so.

When you are in the face-down position, he will probably work round your back with his hands, trying to assess the problem more fully before embarking on actual treatment.

What is osteopathic treatment?

But what exactly is the osteopathic treatment? This obviously isn't a guidebook on how to do osteopathy, so I am not going to describe here how to carry out osteopathic manipulations. Instead, I'm just going to explain what it feels like to be on the receiving end.

My own experience of being treated by many osteopaths is that they combine a process of massaging your aching joints and muscles, plus some stretching movements, with a series of quite dramatic 'thrusts'.

These thrusts are directed at particular joints in the back, and they often produce a loud cracking sound from the spine, accompanied by an astonishing feeling that something has shifted. The first occasion on which this happens to you can be quite alarming. It may also be slightly painful. However, there are times when it produces marked relief in backache.

Very often, these thrusts are directed at your thoracic spine – that is, the section of your spine that lies at the back of your chest. The osteopath gets you to lie face upwards, and puts a small pillow over your breastbone. Next, he turns you slightly, so that he can put one of his hands behind your back. His other hand is on the pillow. Then, he asks you to breathe right out. Suddenly, he thrusts down hard through the pillow. You feel an extraordinary crunching sensation in your backbone. And you will almost certainly need a few seconds to recover, before he moves on to the next joint ...

If you are getting *low* backache, the osteopath will manipulate your lumbar spine – particularly if you have a disc problem in this area. The sort of thing he may do is shown in Figure 6.1, where the osteopath is trying to manipulate the area around the fourth and fifth lumbar vertebrae. This is a very common region for trouble to arise.

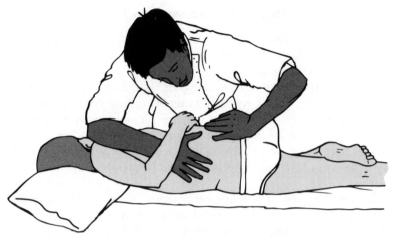

Figure 6.1 Osteopath manipulating lumbar vertebrae

Another common osteopathic manipulation is directed towards the sacro-iliac joint. As we have seen, the S-I joint is located near the top of the buttock, where many people have a dimple in the skin. As I explained earlier in the book, derangement of this joint is an extremely frequent cause of back pain – very often, a dragging kind of ache that is made worse by trying to stand up from a chair.

If the osteopath decides that your S-I joints need manipulating, he will lay you on your side, and arrange your limbs in a precise way. He will then deliver a thrust that goes through the joint. Sometimes you feel a sensation of movement in it, and with luck the pain will ease. In the USA, this manoeuvre is sometimes known as 'the millionaire's roll'.

Osteopaths are also quite likely to use the strength of their arms to stretch out your spine. This is called 'traction', and it often eases pain.

By the time you've finished an osteopathic session, you may well feel a bit drained. In some ways, it's a bit like doing a brisk gym work-out, or three rounds with a boxing coach. So you need to take it easy for an hour or so afterwards, and it may even be a good idea to have someone else drive you home. But please don't sit around immobile. A little gentle exercise is fine.

You might feel a rather 'bruised' sensation on the day after treatment, but that's nothing to be alarmed about.

What fees will you pay?

At the end of the consultation, you'll be asked to pay the fee, since virtually all osteopathic treatment is private in the UK.

I am frequently assured by my patients, or by journalists, that they've heard that osteopathy is available on the NHS these days. In general, this is not true. A very small number of health authorities and hospitals have taken the forward-looking decision to try to provide osteopathic services for those with back pain. However, some of these schemes have 'gone under', owing to lack of funds. So, unless you are very lucky, your osteopathic treatment will be private. How much will you pay?

This varies greatly, depending on whether you go to an expensive practitioner in a posh house in London's Harley Street, or to someone in a low-rent consulting room in a provincial town. In 2008–9, most of the osteopaths I know are charging about £35 for a session, but inflation will of course affect this.

In many cases, it is possible to reclaim your fees from your private health insurance company, but you need to check this *before* you make your appointment.

Will you have to see the osteopath again? Almost certainly. But very often, two or three sessions with him may be enough to get you well on the road to recovery.

None of the osteopaths I've consulted has ever put pressure on me to keep coming back repeatedly.

Osteopathy in various countries

This book describes the situation of osteopathy in the UK, but if you got back trouble while in other countries, could you get osteopathic treatment?

The answer is a qualified 'yes'. There are good osteopaths in Ireland, and also in a number of Commonwealth countries – notably Australia, New Zealand and Canada. In the West Indies, there are a few practising in Barbados, Trinidad and Saint-Barthélemy, but little else.

As for Europe, there are now over 50 registered osteopaths in France – where osteopathy used to be illegal – and there are around 30 in Spain, six in Germany, and a handful in Switzerland. So the osteopathic discipline has not yet spread very widely on the Continent.

In the USA, osteopathy has gone in a totally different direction from the rest of the world. With the American system, there are now many 'osteopathic physicians' or 'doctors of osteopathic medicine' (DOs). These are fully qualified physicians or surgeons who also do some osteopathy. In addition, there are traditional osteopaths, who are not qualified in medicine.

Does osteopathy work?

Opponents of osteopathy often point out that there is a distinct lack of properly controlled trials that prove that osteopathy works. They have a point, but in fact it is almost impossible to organize a rigorous 'double blind' trial of osteopathic treatment. To do this, you would need to set up one group of people, and give them osteopathic manipulation. At the same time, you would have to take a similar group, and give them 'dummy osteopathy' – which would be very difficult. Finally, you would need to ensure that the osteopaths who were doing the treatment didn't know whether they were giving real or 'dummy' osteopathy – which would be absurd.

Both osteopaths and chiropractors point to the findings of the recent UK Back Pain, Exercise and Manipulation study (known as 'UK BEAM'), which seems to indicate that both disciplines give satisfactory results in relieving pain in the lower back.

To be more pragmatic, there are about seven million osteopathic consultations per year in the UK, which suggests that people are satisfied with it, and think that it works. Many report enthusiastically that their backs feel much better after manipulation – though others don't.

Personally, I am aware that when a good osteopath has shifted my spine around, my backache has often been reduced significantly. I appreciate that that's not very scientific evidence! But if I get back pain again, I shall definitely be returning to my excellent local osteopath – or if I'm travelling away from home, perhaps to a chiropractor.

Is osteopathy dangerous?

Opponents of osteopathy – particularly some doctors in the USA – have traditionally attacked it on the grounds that 'osteopaths can really damage you'. Indeed, I have been assured by some conservative American physicians that 'we guys spend a lot of time trying to patch up the harm done by osteopaths'. Frankly, this strikes me as most unlikely. In my entire life, I have never seen someone who has been 'damaged' by an osteopath.

I feel that a useful guide to the safety of osteopathy is this. In the

UK, nearly all health professionals take out some sort of insurance against being sued for 'malpractice' – in other words, if something goes wrong. Surgeons and obstetricians have to pay annual premiums of many thousands of pounds in order to protect themselves against such eventualities.

GPs usually have to pay around £4,000 per annum to their medical defence society to insure themselves against mishaps. But the average osteopath is paying out only about £350 to £400 a year. This really does suggest that osteopathic accidents aren't common at all.

However, any kind of treatment can sometimes go wrong. Very occasionally, one hears of mishaps that have occurred when someone's neck has been vigorously manipulated by a health professional.

More of this in the next chapter – which is on chiropractic.

7

Getting help from a chiropractor

Apart from osteopathy, the other really common 'manipulating' method of getting relief from backache is chiropractic. Its practitioners are called 'chiropractors', and I suppose I must say at the outset that in the UK there is considerable – but discreet – rivalry between them and osteopaths.

Let me affirm my neutrality. Over the years, I have had very good treatment from both chiropractors and osteopaths, and if I ever get pain again I would be happy to go to either type of professional – especially as both disciplines are now properly regulated by law in the UK. Chiropractors have really got their act together – just like the osteopaths – so that they are now run by a statutorily appointed body (the General Chiropractic Council) which maintains a register of trained practitioners. So in the UK, it is no longer possible for any Tom, Dick or Harry to call himself a chiropractor and give you 'quack' treatment for your back.

Confusion between chiropractors, osteopaths and others

Unfortunately, a lot of people with back pain are still very confused about what a chiropractor is. I often see those who tell me that they've 'been to a chiropractor', when in fact they've really gone to an osteopath – or vice versa.

Indeed, there is frequent confusion in the media about what chiropractic is. For instance, at the end of 2007, three normally reliable British newspapers published quite startling articles which stated:

'CHIROPRACTORS ARE A WASTE OF MONEY'

'CHIROPRACTORS ARE A WASTE OF TIME'

'CHIROPRACTORS MAY BE OF NO USE IN TREATING BACK PAIN'

The story was based on a research paper about pain in the lower back that appeared in *The Lancet* that day. However, in reality the *Lancet* report was nothing at all to do with chiropractic. It didn't even mention the word 'chiropractor'.

In fact, the report was about an Australian trial that assessed the merits of the drug diclofenac, compared with physiotherapy. Somehow or other, the journalists had muddled up 15 Australian physiotherapists with British chiropractors. It's not that I am impugning Australian physiotherapists in any way, but simply pointing out what happens when newspapers get the wrong end of the stick.

This kind of glorious misunderstanding is all too common. Some people actually confuse chiropractors with chiropodists! So in this chapter I'm going to explain what chiropractic is – and what it can do for your backache.

Incidentally, if you have started with this chapter, you'll find the main differences between chiropractors and osteopaths are outlined at the beginning of Chapter 6.

What is chiropractic?

So what exactly is chiropractic? Well, the name comes from two Greek words, meaning 'hand' and 'work'. Therefore, chiropractic (*not* 'chiropractice') means that the practitioner works on your body with her hands. There is no use of drugs, nor surgery either.

And that's really the main thing that chiropractors do: they try to make your backache better by using their fingers and palms on it. (It is a curious coincidence that the founder of chiropractic was a chap called 'Palmer'.) They do try to treat other conditions apart from backache, but those are outside the scope of this book.

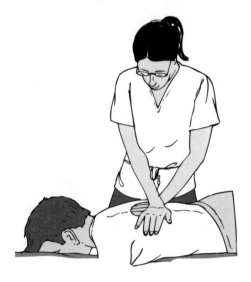

Figure 7.1 Chiropractor adjusting client's back

All of this may sound very like osteopathy to you, but in fact the manipulations (or, as chiropractors call them, 'adjustments') are rather different. Chiropractic professionals tend to use them directly on or near the problem areas of your back, in contrast to osteopathic manipulations which are often carried out by levering or thrusting on some other part of the body.

In Figure 7.1, you can see the way that chiropractors use their hands directly on your back.

But to the average person on the couch, the two types of treatment may feel much the same – or, at least, that has been my own experience. For instance, both chiropractic and osteopathy often involve working on spinal joints in a way that produces a loud 'click' or crunch. This is usually very satisfying to the person on the couch – and maybe to the practitioner as well. Fortunately, it is sometimes followed by a reduction in pain – though that isn't always so.

This noise is rather like the sort of thing you may well have heard when you give someone you love a really big hug, or if they put their arms around your chest and squeeze you firmly. What causes it? Well, a lot of manipulators say that it's due to the 'popping' of a bubble in the fluid of a joint. If you search the internet, you'll find that this is often referred to as an 'air bubble', but that is quite impossible. We do *not* have air forming in our joints. But it could be carbon dioxide, which is present in joint fluid, or possibly nitrogen.

As far as I can discover, the claim that bubbles cause the sound is based on research done in 1947 and 1971 by two groups of doctors who X-rayed people's hands while they 'cracked' their own knuckles. The 1947 group of medics thought that the noise was caused by the *formation* of a bubble in the knuckle joint, while the 1971 group said that it was caused by the bubble *bursting*. No one has ever demonstrated any bubbles popping in the spinal column.

When I've been on the receiving end of a chiropractor's adjustment of my spine, the 'crunch' has sounded much more like two bones moving – as if an out-of-place joint was being moved. Be that as it may, chiropractors, like osteopaths, certainly do manage to make *something* happen in your spine. And, quite often, this 'something' is followed by relief of pain.

Dr James Cyriax dismissed the whole issue by saying that the noise could be due to 'all sorts of things' – including perhaps a disc going back into place.

In a moment, we'll discuss what actually happens when you go to a chiropractor. But first, can I just explain the curious but interesting history of chiropractic.

History of chiropractic

Chiropractic was invented by a Canadian called Daniel Palmer, who coined the term while working in America in 1895. About a year later, he opened a school of chiropractic in Davenport, Iowa.

Therefore Palmer developed the idea of chiropractic just a couple of years after Andrew Still started up the first college of osteopathy in Kirksville, Missouri.

Did the two men know each other? History is silent on that point. However, while researching this book I checked some maps of the USA and found to my astonishment that the two colleges were in fact only 140 miles (224 km) from each other. Also, there were excellent transport services between Kirksville and Davenport including the famous Wabash Railroad – and, for part of the way, the Mississippi River steamboats. At that time, you could easily cover the distance between the home of osteopathy and the home of chiropractic in a day or so.

Isn't that remarkable? The two biggest 'complementary' systems of medicine in the whole of the Western world started life just a hop and a skip down the road from each other. So it's almost impossible to imagine that this pair of 'founding fathers' didn't know about each other's work.

Indeed, while delving into the history of chiropractic I was interested to note that in the mid-1890s there was a chap called Andrew Davis – a qualified doctor – who studied at the new osteopathic college in Kirksville, and then moved up the Mississippi to join Daniel Palmer's chiropractic college in Davenport. After being there a short while, he published a book on *osteopathy*. That must have confused people a bit ...

Clearly, then, the origins of chiropractic and osteopathy were closely linked. In particular, both Still and Palmer had a basic belief that adjustment of the spine could cure not only backache, but also a multitude of illnesses elsewhere in the body.

What is also obvious is that both of them knew about what the old bone-setters of the Mid-West could do, with their skill at repairing damaged cowboys (and others) by means of 'cracking' joints. I suspect that they must also have been aware of the skills of the 'medicine men' of the native American tribes.

Just like osteopathy, chiropractic was sneered at by the American medical establishment, and particularly by orthodox doctors in the town of Davenport – who doubtless saw it as a threat to their trade. Attempts were made to prosecute chiropractors for 'practicing medicine without a license'. But Daniel Palmer carried on, despite insults and threats of legal action.

To begin with, he called his chiropractic establishment 'The School of Magnetic Medicine', because he believed that he had special magnetic powers in his hands that could help him detect areas of inflammation in his clients. He also thought that he could make inflamed tissue better by putting his own vital magnetism into it. However, as the years went by, the idea of magnetic therapy was quietly dropped.

In 1895–6, Palmer managed to improve the deafness of his janitor by manipulating a 'displacement' in his neck. As a result of that success, for a few years he taught that these displacements in the spine caused 'inflammation' elsewhere in the body.

There was also a good deal of inflammation of another kind among the nearby Missouri osteopaths. They accused Daniel Palmer of being 'a thief' who had stolen large chunks of osteopathy, and was selling it to the public as 'chiropractic'.

It may have been partly because of those attacks by osteopaths that he changed his theory of disease. In 1902, Palmer decided that displacements in the spinal bones actually affected the health of the rest of the body by pressing on *nerves*. This was the so-called 'bone pinches nerve' theory, which has tended to underpin chiropractic ever since.

By 1903, Palmer had decided that 95 per cent of all human diseases were caused by subluxations (i.e. minor displacements) in the spinal joints that were pressing on nerves. He had already declared that 'injury to certain nerves' was a cause of cancer, and that he could cure it by adjusting the spine.

In 1906, Palmer was jailed for 23 days on a manifestly unfair charge of practising medicine without a licence. Undeterred, he continued working – and came up with other theories of why his system of treatment worked. However, they have now been almost forgotten by the chiropractic profession.

Thanks to the efforts of his son, Bartlett Palmer, it was the 'bone pinches nerve' idea that gradually spread across America and a number of other countries – helped by the fact that chiropractors were undeniably successful in treating backache.

Chiropractic reached Britain after the First World War, and in 1925 the British Chiropractic Association was formed, with just six members. Despite this, very few people in the UK had heard of chiropractic until quite late in the twentieth century. When I was first researching back pain in the 1970s, it was extremely difficult to find a qualified chiropractor in many parts of the country. That has now changed, largely thanks to the establishment of the well-known Anglo-European College of Chiropractic in Bournemouth. This provides a four-year degree course, and it currently graduates about 90 practitioners a year – a figure that will increase rapidly in the near future.

However, even today chiropractors are heavily outnumbered by osteopaths, who have about 4,000 practitioners, as opposed to the chiropractic profession's 2,500. But in most parts of the UK today, you won't have any trouble finding a chiropractor.

Although chiropractic has been statutorily regulated in the UK since the Chiropractors Act of 1994, there are in fact three groups of chiropractors. The biggest, with 1,400 members, is the long-established British Chiropractic Association, which only accepts people who have graduated from a nationally recognized college of chiropractic education, such as the Bournemouth college.

A smaller group are called 'the McTimoney chiropractors'. Their headquarters are based at Abingdon, in Oxfordshire, and they now have over 500 practitioners, located mainly in central and southern England. They're still very thin on the ground in some areas, notably Scotland.

The origin of this particular type of chiropractic is a rather interesting story. In 1942, an English technical illustrator called John McTimoney was treated for back pain by a Mr Ashford – who had learned chiropractic long ago in America under Daniel Palmer. Because of McTimoney's interest in the way mechanical things worked, he became fascinated by the idea of chiropractic, and towards the end of the Second World War he made contact with an American-trained manipulator called Mary Walker. She taught him and another Briton how to manipulate, and he finally qualified as a 'Doctor of Chiropractic' in 1950.

As a technically minded man, McTimoney started developing chiropractic techniques of his own – notably something called 'the toggle-torque recoil', which is a way of manipulating the neck. Alas, he then developed cardiac problems. In 1972, wishing to ensure the continuation of his work after his death, he opened the Oxfordshire School of Chiropractic. Before he died in 1980, he managed to train 14 'disciples'. Nowadays, the School has become the McTimoney College of Chiropractic at Abingdon, which awards its BSc to about 70 students a year.

For a while, the McTimoney graduates were definitely looked down on by 'mainstream' chiropractors, partly because some of their training was by postal tuition. However, these days they – like the British Chiropractic Association members – are on the Register of Chiropractors. Interestingly, some of them have branched out into giving chiropractic to small animals and horses.

The third training organization is a more recently established one: the Welsh Institute of Chiropractic, which is located at Treforest, near Pontypridd. This is part of the University of Glamorgan, and currently it is producing around 70 qualified chiropractors per year. Unusually, it has its own MRI scanner.

Personally, I only have experience of being treated by chiropractors who are members of the British Chiropractic Association. However, my researches for this book have made me feel that anyone who is on the General Chiropractic Register could be worth talking to when you have bad backache.

So if you are travelling somewhere in the UK or Ireland and are suddenly struck by back pain, it's not a bad idea to look in the *Yellow Pages* (or *Golden Pages* in Ireland) to see if there is a registered chiropractor in the area. To check if someone is on the Register, ring the General Chiropractic Council or visit their website (see Useful addresses at the back of this book).

What happens when you go to a chiropractor?

So let's assume that you've made an appointment with a chiropractor. You walk into her reception room – or perhaps *limp* in, if your back is bad. What happens next?

My experience has been that chiropractors do their level best to be friendly and welcoming, and to make you comfortable. One of the first 'chiros' I visited had a splendid reception area, with lots of comfy sofas. When I arrived there, I was immediately put in a big armchair and shown a couple of videos about chiropractic, explaining what it is, and what benefits it could bring. Curiously, these videos had been made in New Zealand.

I noted that in the videos there was considerable stress on the idea that regular visits to a chiropractor throughout life would be good for your health, and that the whole family could benefit from such regular appointments. We will return to this feature of chiropractic in a moment.

What happens next? Well, when you go in to see the chiropractor you will almost certainly find – as I did – that she is unhurried and very willing to listen to what you have to say. Most chiropractors want to know all about your lifestyle, including what you eat and whether you smoke or drink – as well as what you do in the course of your work, and what sports or hobbies you go in for.

After that, you'll be asked to disrobe. Exactly as is the case with an osteopathic examination, you should undress to your underwear. Men can keep on their underpants, and women their bras and pants. You should be offered a dressing gown or a hospital-style gown. I once encountered a rather bogus manipulator – *not* a registered chiropractor –

who got all his female clients to take their bras off. It should go without saying that this sort of 'manipulator' should be avoided at all costs.

The chiropractor will examine your back thoroughly, in much the same way as I described in Chapter 5. Then you'll be asked to lie on the couch. Chiropractors' couches are often divided into numerous separate movable padded sections, and they do tend to be very agreeable and restful to relax on.

Then the practitioner will set to work on your back with her hands. A lot of people are afraid that this will hurt, but I would rate it as generally a pleasant experience – though you may experience minor discomfort (and surprise) during certain adjustments of the spine.

What are these 'adjustments'? Well, once again, this isn't a guidebook on how to perform chiropractic. It's actually a guide to how you – the person receiving treatment – will *feel* during the various adjustments. There are apparently at least a hundred different ways of adjusting your back, including such complex techniques as the following:

- Diversified adjusting. This means giving a quick thrust to the spine. It is often accompanied by a loud 'pop'.
- Gonstead technique. This is a way of adjusting your spine, guided by the appearances in your X-rays.
- Sacro-occipital technique. This is an approach in which blocks are placed under your pelvis, while the practitioner gently manipulates your spine. Some chiropractors claim that this 'improves the flow of fluid up and down your spinal cord'.
- Cox flexion distraction. A way of stretching the spine, to relieve backache.
- Nimmo technique. This is a method of applying finger pressure to tender spots in your back, to try to ease the spasm in your muscles.
- Logan technique. This involves prolonged pressure at the base of your spine, to try to correct the alignment of the rest of it.

Also, don't be surprised if your chiropractor produces a slim metal rod, about 15 cm (6 in) long, and applies it to your back. This is called an 'Activator', and it's a device that she uses to try to resolve spinal problems, by pressing the end against your vertebrae. It is *not* an instrument of torture, and it shouldn't hurt you.

Many of the above are quite gentle adjustments, from the point of view of the person on the receiving end. However, my advice to you is to *ask* the chiropractor what she's going to do, before she actually embarks on it. Among the few criticisms I've heard of chiropractic is the suggestion that sometimes practitioners do a high-speed thrust, and 'pop' your spine before you realize what is about to happen. However, they are supposed to warn you first.

Personally, the only things that I have found at all alarming about chiropractic manipulation are the techniques that they may use on your neck. This book is about backache, not neck disorders. However, please note that if you are also having neck problems, chiropractors may – after, I hope, giving you due warning – put their fingers firmly on your neck, and then give you a sudden and quite dramatic twist.

I have always found that this quick 'torque' on the neck region of my spine comes as a bit of a psychological shock, especially as it is usually accompanied by loud noises from the cervical vertebrae. Indeed, these neck twists have caused some controversy – see below.

For completeness, I should add that a similar procedure is done by osteopaths in cases of neck pain and stiffness.

At the end of the physical part of your session, the practitioner might well suggest an X-ray, as an aid to diagnosis. This is quite a contrast with family doctors, who are very reluctant to X-ray backs these days, partly because of the slight risks of radiation – and partly because imaging departments refuse to comply with the GP's request, on the grounds that an X-ray wouldn't show anything useful.

Some 120 British chiropractic clinics actually have an X-ray machine on the premises. The others will probably refer you to the radiography departments of local private clinics or hospitals if they feel you need an X-ray.

Also, it is very likely that the chiropractor will finish by giving you advice about your lifestyle, including your physical activities and perhaps your diet. A lot of this advice is likely to be worth heeding, if you want to avoid further episodes of backache. She may also give you exercises to do at home, and will probably advise you about your seating (at home, at work and in the car).

Does chiropractic work?

Does chiropractic treatment work? From my own experience, I would say that it often does – though sometimes it doesn't.

Admittedly, once again, that's not a very scientific assessment. But as I explained in the chapter on osteopathy, it is very difficult to do a valid, rigidly controlled clinical trial of a system of manipulation. However, chiropractors in the UK feel that there have been trials that back up their claims that their treatment can be beneficial in cases of backache. The College of Chiropractors quotes the following:

- Medical Research Council trials, which were published in the *British Medical Journal* in 1990 and 1995, which found that

chiropractic was substantially better than hospital out-patient treatment for chronic, severe pain in the lower back.
- The UK BEAM Trial, published in the *British Medical Journal* in 2004, which showed that both exercise and 'manipulation' helped those with back pain to recover better.

This is not exactly evidence of chiropractic being a miracle cure, but then nothing else provides miraculous cures for back pain, does it? And when I see people with backache who have been to a chiropractor, and who report that they felt 'much less pain' after having their spines adjusted, then I am inclined to give chiropractic the benefit of the doubt.

Yes ... I know that it could all be a placebo effect. But it's certainly worth trying.

Are there any dangers?

Once you start researching chiropractic, you suddenly find that there is a curious amount of virulent hostility to it, particularly in countries like New Zealand and Canada. I didn't find it easy to discover why there was all this antagonism.

After a while, I realized that some people are against chiropractic because they say that 'it opposes immunization' for various illnesses. That has certainly been true of the American and Canadian chiropractic professions in the past. But in the UK it doesn't seem to be so; the British Chiropractic Association tell me that they 'have no position on immunization'.

Eventually I discovered that a lot of anti-chiropractic sentiment has arisen because a number of people claim to have been injured by chiropractic manipulation. In particular, there are frequent attacks on the type of 'sudden neck twist' manoeuvre used by chiropractors, which (so it is alleged) can actually cause a stroke.

The suggestion by opponents of chiropractic is that the rapid movement can tear through the vertebral arteries – which run upwards through the cervical vertebrae to supply the brain. If you want to read more, have a look at one of several extremely angry websites that are administered by anti-chiropractic factions. The British one is run by 'Action for Victims of Chiropractic' (<www.chirovictims.org.uk>).

I put my concerns about strokes to the British Chiropractic Association, and they replied, through their PR company: 'People may seek treatment from a chiropractor ... due to pre-stroke symptoms such as headache or neck pain, so there may be a small association between having a chiropractic treatment and then suffering a stroke, but this does not imply causation.'

One well-known American chiropractor, Gary Farr, says: 'Based on published cases and insurance reports, complications from genuine chiropractic manipulation to the neck are, at worst, a problem for one in 500,000 patients. That's just 0.0002 per cent.'

Furthermore, the General Chiropractic Council has drawn my attention to a fairly convincing piece of research from Ontario, which seems to show that the risk of a stroke after chiropractic treatment is virtually the same as the risk after seeing a GP. And various chiropractors have told me they feel that people who were about to have a stroke might get a headache and therefore consult a chiropractor, or a doctor, just beforehand.

I take no sides in this matter. However, if you are going to go to a chiropractor for treatment of backache, then obviously you should be aware that such accusations exist. That is particularly important if you are planning to have neck manipulation as well. Some chiropractic clinics specifically state on their websites that they do *not* do the controversial neck manipulation.

Claims that chiropractic can damage the *back* – as opposed to the neck – are rare. And I must add that personally I have never seen a person who has been harmed by a chiropractor.

Finally, I pointed out in the last chapter that the sums that osteopaths have to pay in insurance each year are small, in comparison with those paid out by doctors and surgeons. This clearly implies that medics are more likely to damage you than osteopaths are!

Much the same applies to the chiropractic profession. According to the British Chiropractic Association, the average chiropractor only has to contribute £500 to £700 per annum to protect herself against legal action. In contrast, as mentioned earlier, the average GP has to pay about £4,000 per annum.

Therefore, you can see that a doctor is much more likely to be sued than a chiropractor is.

A question of fees

So what are you likely to pay if you decide to go to a chiropractor because of back pain? Fees vary greatly. For instance:

- One clinic in the 'finance district' of the City of London currently charges £130 for an initial consultation.
- One on the edge of south-west London charges £49.
- One on the Sussex coast makes no charge for the initial consultation, but charges £45 for a subsequent examination.

Please bear in mind that X-rays of your back cost extra, and will be anything from £22 to £60 per plate.

These fees may seem fairly high, especially if you're short of cash. However, it is still possible to find a chiropractor who charges only £25 a session. Also, quite a few chiropractic clinics make a habit of advertising 'special offers' in the local press – sometimes with a free initial session.

Also, if you belong to a private health scheme, such as BUPA or PPP, you may find that your policy covers chiropractic treatment. Please note that some policies require you to get a referral letter from your GP. (*Important*: make sure that the chiropractor you choose is actually registered with your health insurance scheme.)

I'm afraid that contrary to what many people believe, chiropractic is only rarely available through the NHS. That may change as the years go by.

Signing up for a long-term course of chiropractic treatment

One slightly puzzling thing about chiropractic is that some practitioners want you to sign up for long-term treatment.

This does not tend to happen with osteopaths, physiotherapists or doctors.

For instance, the leaflet of one London clinic offers you a course of 36 adjustments for £1,080. The thinking behind these schemes seems to be that chiropractic is something that you (and maybe your family) should have *for life* – with regular spinal treatment every few weeks.

The General Chiropractic Council has recently warned the public against paying in advance for a year's therapy. As they rightly say: 'Why would you need a year's treatment? How does the chiropractor know in advance that you need a year's treatment? Will you get a full refund if you decide to discontinue treatment?'

I agree with the General Chiropractic Council. Unless you really need long-term therapy for your backache, and are being offered a substantial discount, it seems foolish to pay for more than one session at a time.

Summing up

The scientific evidence for the effectiveness of chiropractic in treating backache is really no better than the fairly modest evidence for the effectiveness of osteopathy. But even though it *is* modest, it exists.

Huge numbers of people who have backache are prepared to swear that 'the chiropractor really helped me'. So if your doctor cannot put your back right, it is certainly worth your while trying chiropractic.

And now we move on ... to physiotherapy.

8

Getting help from a physiotherapist

Physiotherapists can help you with your backache. They have been part of the UK medical scene – and of the 'back-pain scene' – for well over one hundred years. And you find them in most Commonwealth countries too. However, in some parts of the world – notably the USA – they are known as 'physical therapists'. If you are a devotee of the wonderful TV series *Frasier*, you'll have often heard that description applied to Daphne Moon. Indeed, these days physiotherapists are often known in the UK and other countries as 'PTs'.

Physiotherapists are also found in France and western Europe, where they are usually called 'kinés' – which is short for *kinésithérapeutes*. In German-speaking countries they are known as *Heilgymnasten*.

What does a physiotherapist do?

What do they do? Well, the Chartered Society of Physiotherapy explains their work like this:

- using physical approaches to promote, maintain and restore well-being;
- being science-based;
- exercising clinical judgement and informed interpretation of your signs and symptoms.

OK, but what can they actually *do* for your painful back?

Well, the fact is that they are *not* going to claim to cure it with some magic remedy. I have never heard a physiotherapist say 'I cured his back.' Indeed, I've usually found them to be modest people, who make moderate claims that are – where possible – supported by scientific evidence.

In general, what they aim to achieve is:

- to ease your pain;
- to increase your mobility;
- to help you get back to work and/or your other usual activities.

They manage this by using a selection of the following approaches:

- massage;

- manipulation;
- mobilization;
- exercises;
- electrical therapy;
- education and advice;
- traction (rare these days in the UK);
- ultrasound.

History of physiotherapy

Since earliest times, people have been aware that one human being can often help another by applying soothing hands to a painful area of the body, so massage and manipulation have in that sense been practised for many hundreds of years.

When did all this develop into physiotherapy? Oddly enough, it began at almost exactly the same time as the osteopaths and the chiropractors were setting up their first colleges in the American Mid-West. It seems that in the 1890s, the world was in the right mood for physical therapy.

In England, the start of physiotherapy came in 1894 when a young nurse called Lucy Robinson, together with three of her friends, set up the Society of Trained Masseuses. Their objective was to prevent the profession of medical massage 'falling into disrepute'. Yes, even in those days there were quite a lot of ladies who were offering an entirely different type of massage ...

Soon after that, a number of British teaching hospitals founded 'Schools of Massage'. These new schools not only provided hands-on therapy, but also something called 'Medical Gymnastics'. Electrical treatments and special baths were usually provided, and some experts in physical medicine were imported from Sweden.

Similar progress was made in the Commonwealth and in the USA, where the Walter Reed Hospital started employing women who were known as 'Reconstruction Aides'.

During the First World War, there was an explosion of need for these health workers – to treat the wounded. In 1921, Mary McMillan set up what is now the American Physical Therapy Association (APTA). The APTA remains the leading US organization in this field.

All over the world from the 1920s onwards, more and more physiotherapists were required, because of the terrible poliomyelitis epidemics that paralysed so many people, leaving them with wasted muscles and often great difficulties in breathing. These outbreaks lasted until the late 1950s (when use of polio vaccine became widespread), and physiotherapists played a vital part in helping the survivors.

In Britain, the Society of Trained Masseuses changed its name a few times, but in 1944 it became the Chartered Society of Physiotherapy (CSP). The title 'physiotherapist' is now protected in law, which means that frauds/quacks can no longer claim that they are physiotherapists. (However, beware: there are people who advertise themselves with words that *sound* a bit like 'physiotherapist' – for instance, 'physiologist'.)

Nowadays, the Chartered Society of Physiotherapy represents a staggering 47,000 members in the UK. So there are considerably more physiotherapists than there are GPs, and there are ten times as many physiotherapists as osteopaths.

Therefore, in the UK, there is a massive 'resource' of physiotherapists who could help you with your backache. This chapter will tell you how to make use of them.

Getting to see a physiotherapist

In physiotherapy, one important change has slowly taken place. For many decades, the physiotherapists were very much 'under the thumb' of the doctors, so you could only take your bad back to a physiotherapist if your doctor agreed.

I don't think this was a good situation at all. I can clearly remember when the medical profession used to issue orders to physiotherapists as to how they should treat patients. Quite often, these orders were given by silly young medics – including myself – who knew much less about physical medicine than the physiotherapists did.

Things are different now. Since 1977, members of the Chartered Society of Physiotherapy have been able to treat back pain and other conditions *without* first receiving a referral letter from a doctor.

However, in effect this only applied to private medicine, and not to the NHS. Certainly, a lot of physiotherapists now run private clinics, to which you can go without a doctor's letter. (There are about 4,000 private physiotherapists.) You can find these clinics listed in your local *Yellow Pages* under 'Physiotherapists' – look for the large box headed 'Chartered Physiotherapists'.

Nevertheless, within the NHS, the same old rigid system has continued. If you want physiotherapy on the NHS, generally you still need to go to your GP first, and persuade her to send a referral form to the local hospital's Physiotherapy Department.

But I'm glad to report that a big change is taking place in the UK. A new scheme is gradually being introduced, in which people will be able to go to NHS physiotherapists *direct* – without the intervention of a GP. This 'self-referral' project is largely dependent on local agreements, so it may or may not get started soon in your area. In Scotland, it has already begun.

One variant of it is going to be 'triage' (sorting) over the phone by the physiotherapist. In other words, you ring up the physiotherapist and tell her your symptoms, and she then decides whether it would be worth your while coming into her department for treatment.

But for the moment, the reality is that most people who have backache will go initially to a GP. If she can't 'get you right' within, say, a month or so, then the question of having some physiotherapy has to be considered. If you would like to try it, and if your GP agrees, then she will write out a request and send it off to the Physiotherapy Department.

However, there remains one big problem – the delays of the NHS. The average person naturally assumes that if his GP refers him for physiotherapy because of backache, he might be seen within a week or so. I'm afraid that in many areas of the country, that just isn't true. Regrettably, I have had people complain to me that they have been waiting anything up to three and a half months for a physiotherapy appointment. In some cases, the back pain gets better before they receive an appointment.

On the other hand, there are now some parts of the UK (notably Scotland) where general practices actually have an 'attached' physiotherapist, who will see you very promptly.

But if the waiting times are long in your area, and if you can afford to pay for treatment, it may perhaps be worth considering going to a physiotherapist privately.

What to expect when you see a physiotherapist

Whether you're seeing a physiotherapist privately or on the NHS, she will be a highly trained professional. She will treat you with respect, and she will do her best for your back problem.

When you go for your appointment, she will invariably take a careful 'history' of the important facts connected with your backache – like how long you've had it, whether anything started it off, whether anything makes it worse, and whether anything makes it better.

She should also ask you about your work, your hobbies, your sports – and your medication. She will probably be interested in what sort of chairs you sit in – at work, at home, and in the car. She will then examine you carefully.

However, from then on, it is a little hard to forecast precisely what she will do. This is because different physiotherapists have very different ways of dealing with back pain.

The three professions that we've already considered up to now in the book (medicine, osteopathy and chiropractic) possess fairly clearly defined schemes of treatment. With physiotherapists, it is a little different. Much depends on the protocols laid down by the department or clinic in which they work. Also, individual physiotherapists tend to be influenced by the styles of treatment that were used in their own training school.

Overall, though, it's likely that the therapy that the physiotherapist gives you will involve one or more of the types of treatment listed in the next section.

Types of physiotherapy treatment

An important thing to appreciate about physiotherapy is that it isn't just *one* type of treatment.

'Physio' is completely unlike any other discipline in that it includes an extraordinary and diverse range of physical therapies, which have somehow got incorporated into it as the years have gone by. Many of these therapies have absolutely nothing in common with one another. Some of them are not used by many practitioners these days, while others remain very popular.

Occasionally, I see those who say to me 'I tried physio for my backache last Thursday, but it obviously doesn't work. So I never bothered going along for the second appointment.'

This is very short-sighted. There are well over a dozen different methods of treatment that are used by physiotherapists these days, and it's unwise to assume that 'physio doesn't work' when you've only tried one type.

Massage

As you have a back pain, the physiotherapist will almost certainly lay you face-down on a couch and give you some form of back massage with her hands. The type of massage varies quite a lot, but my own experience has been that physiotherapists are very good at soothing aching muscles with their fingers and palms. And when the musculature has gone into spasm – which is often the case in backache – they can make it relax once more.

Manipulation

Physiotherapists are nowhere near as involved in manipulation as, say, osteopaths are, and some physiotherapists do no manipulating at all. However, depending on her training, your therapist might well offer you some manipulation of your back. Specialist physiotherapists can be very good at this.

There are two systems of manipulation that are particularly associated with physiotherapy, and they are called 'Cyriax' and 'Maitland'.

Cyriax

As mentioned earlier in the book, Cyriax manipulation is named after the great English physician Dr James Cyriax, who treated me with it on many occasions. It is often used by physiotherapy graduates from his old hospital, St Thomas', in London. Basically, it is a system of using the operator's thumb-tips to work up and down the spine, pressing directly inwards. Personally, I have found that it often gives considerable relief from pain.

I have an abiding memory of feeling a lot better at the end of one session at a London hospital, and then hearing my formidable physiotherapist remark to her colleague: 'Righto! You take over, Vera. I've just Cyriaxed him ...'!

Dr Cyriax did also develop a lot of other manipulation techniques – directed at various specific joints – and these are used by some physiotherapists.

Maitland

Maitland manipulation is named after a brilliant Australian physiotherapist, Geoffrey Maitland. In the 1960s, he had the good sense to make an extensive study of the manipulative systems used by other physiotherapists, by osteopaths, by chiropractors and by medical doctors (including Cyriax).

Eventually, he developed his own system, which involves a detailed manual examination of the person's spine, thus – one hopes – leading to accurate diagnosis. This is followed by precise therapy, tailored to each individual's needs. The treatment includes:

- manual adjustment of the vertebrae;
- manual joint mobilization;
- manual stretching of muscles;
- training in posture;
- exercises specific to the problem.

One of the strengths of Maitland's method is that he constantly used 'feedback' from the person – adjusting his therapy according to how the man or woman reacted. Today, the Maitland method – or, as its adherents prefer to call it, 'the Maitland Concept' – is taught all over the Western world, and especially in Australia and the rest of the Commonwealth.

Exercises

We've mentioned exercise quite a bit in this chapter and earlier ones. Physiotherapists quite rightly lay special emphasis on the value of exercises. These can be things that you do in the Physiotherapy Department/Clinic, and also exercises that the physiotherapist gives you to do at home.

It's very worthwhile following her 'exercise prescription'. Research suggests that exercise is one of the most effective aspects of physiotherapy, and failure to take exercise is notoriously bad for backache.

Hydrotherapy

Hydrotherapy is essentially doing exercises in water. The water takes the weight off your back, and makes it easier for you to use your back muscles. It should be pleasantly warm! With luck, muscular spasm is relieved and pain reduced.

Some fortunate Physiotherapy Departments have their own hydrotherapy baths or access to swimming pools. Using these is very soothing for backache. However, avoid doing the breaststroke, as this puts a surprising amount of strain on the upper spine, especially the neck.

Electrical therapy

For the best part of 200 years, doctors, therapists, masseuses and downright quacks have tried to use electricity to treat back pain and other problems. You see, people were usually very impressed by electricity – especially if it made buzzing noises or flashes or explosions, and gave you minor shocks. In the first half of the twentieth century, incredibly intricate and dramatic-looking electrical apparatus was used on people with backache. If you look at the electricity room at the Harrogate health spa in the film *Agatha*, starring Vanessa Redgrave, which is about the 'walkabout period' in Agatha Christie's life, you'll see what I mean.

In reality, electrical treatment is a bit limited in its medical uses. However, physiotherapists do employ it to relieve pain, and to try to help healing by increasing blood flow in the affected area.

For instance, they use electrical TENS machines – which we'll discuss more fully in Chapter 10 – to ease the pain of backache and other conditions. The initials TENS stand for 'Transcutaneous Electrical Nerve Stimulation'. These devices work pretty well on many people, but not on others. As well as employing them in their clinics, physiotherapists often 'lend out' TENS machines to people to use at home.

Also, many Physiotherapy Departments use an electrical system that you'll hear described as 'The Interferential' or 'Interferential Therapy'. This involves passing two electrical currents through your tissues. Don't worry – it doesn't hurt. Where the currents meet, they 'interfere' with each other. The resulting reaction in your tissues is believed to increase blood flow, reduce inflammation, and relieve pain.

Short-wave diathermy (SWD) is a way of producing heat in the tissues – please see below. In the UK, it's no longer much used.

Ultrasound

For about the last 45 years, physiotherapists have used high-pitched sound waves ('ultrasound') on painful areas of the body. These are the same sort of ultrasonic waves that are employed in the course of gynaecology and obstetrics to scan the womb and adjoining organs. But the type of ultrasound used in physiotherapy is intended to make the tissues in your back vibrate imperceptibly. This improves the blood flow to the area, and is thought to speed up healing.

Laser therapy

Many people have an almost mystical belief in laser treatment – even though they may not be quite sure what a laser actually *is*. I've heard someone ask a surgeon to do her operation with a laser, rather than a scalpel, in the belief that things would somehow be far better that way. (The surgeon refused.)

In fact, a laser is just a very pure form of light. The letters stand for 'Light Amplification by Stimulated Emission of Radiation'. It's the sort of thing you have in your DVD player, where the laser is used to 'read' the disc.

Some physiotherapists do use lasers, but I find it hard to see what the beam could do for your backache. However, it is claimed that it's possible to use the tip of the laser beam to carry out a sort of acupuncture (see Chapter 11) on your back.

Traction

Traction means drawing the spinal bones apart. Quite often, doing this eases the pain of back problems. There doesn't seem to be any strong scientific evidence that it works, but those who have just had it will often walk away saying: 'Thanks – I feel quite a lot better.' However, traction has become less popular in recent years, partly because it can occasionally make pain worse instead of better.

The fact that traction does sometimes help is the reason why there are various DIY spine-stretching devices on the market (see Chapter 9). It's also the reason why osteopaths, doctors and chiropractors might take hold of, say, your legs or your head and pull on them firmly.

Some physiotherapists still have the old-fashioned kind of traction apparatus that can draw your vertebrae apart, and they may be worth a try. The two types of apparatus of which I have most experience of being stretched on are:

- The traction bed. This is a bit like the stretching couch that was featured in the James Bond film *Thunderball* (1965), but not in its 1983 remake *Never Say Never Again*. You lie down on it, and are then strapped to it. After that, the physiotherapist turns a handle, or presses a button, making both the top half of the bed and the bottom half gently move apart. As you can imagine, this stretches your spine considerably. Although the principle is rather like that of the medieval torture rack, I never found it painful – and it did sometimes help.
- The head traction apparatus. This is a bit like a cyclist's helmet or scrum cap, to the top of which is attached a cord. The cord runs over a pulley-wheel, and the physiotherapist attaches weights to the end of it. The result is that your upper spine (and particularly the cervical part of it) is stretched.

Heat

As almost everybody knows, heat generally relieves pain. So physiotherapists will often use heat pads, heat 'wraps' and similar devices, which they apply to your spine and adjoining regions.

'Short-wave diathermy' (SWD) treatment is a way of raising the temperature in your tissues, by using an oscillating electrical current of extremely high frequency. So it heats up the area where you have pain. Once popular, it's now only rarely used in the UK.

The effect of heat is only going to be short-lasting. But if it's reasonably effective, you'll then be advised about how to apply heat at home.

Ice

Paradoxically, *cold* can also be helpful for backache. That's why your physiotherapist may apply ice to your skin – usually very near to the site of the back pain. She will also advise you how to use ice or a 'cold pack' at home.

But please take care that you don't injure your skin by putting the pack on unwrapped. In general, anything cold should be wrapped in a towel or a purpose-made cover.

Going privately: costs

There are many private physiotherapy clinics which have sprung up since the profession was freed from the control of doctors, back in 1977. Their charges vary enormously. Here are some examples I have noticed:

- An establishment in the Home Counties, which claims to feature 'the most highly qualified and experienced holistic physiotherapist in the UK', charges £120 for a 90-minute session.
- A Mayfair physiotherapy clinic will charge you £70 for the first half-hour.
- A pleasant clinic on Brighton sea front offers discounted sessions at a cost of £35.
- A consulting room in a working-class district of Glasgow will give people with backache a session at a 'sale offer' price of £30.

(*Important*: Please bear in mind that 'special' treatments, like ultrasound or laser acupuncture, are often listed under 'extra charges'.)

Personally, I have found that physiotherapists are generally very fair in their charging and don't attempt any kind of 'hard sell'. However, you should be just a little careful about signing up for physiotherapy sessions that are really administered by big businesses, like large leisure clubs or private hospitals. Check the list of fees first.

For instance, I clearly remember an occasion when I was in a posh clinic, recovering from an operation. The door of my room was pushed open, and a physiotherapist stuck her head inside. She said: 'I expect you know the post-op exercises, don't you?' I nodded. Then she withdrew her head and was never seen again. This service eventually appeared on my bill as: 'physiotherapist's visit ... £20'. I did not pay.

In practice, many private physiotherapy bills can be reclaimed from private health insurers, such as BUPA or WPA. But check the wording of your policy before you have the treatment – and (most importantly) make sure that your physiotherapist is registered with your medical insurance company.

Also, check to see how many sessions of physiotherapy you are entitled to.

Does physiotherapy work?

As you can see, physiotherapy doesn't claim to be a 'magic cure' for backache. But I'm in no doubt at all that a good physiotherapist can ease your pain and stiffness, and help you to get on with your life.

However, it is difficult to assess all physiotherapeutic treatments scientifically – partly because there are so many of them.

For example, the rigorous Steer Report, carried out by Dr Colin Fischbacher on behalf of the Wessex Institute, found that 'no conclusions can currently be drawn about the effectiveness of a physiotherapy service without paying close attention to the *mix* of treatment methods provided'. All he was able to conclude was that physiotherapy exercises seemed likely to help chronic (i.e. long-term) pain, while keeping the person active seemed to be of use in acute pain.

Nevertheless, if I ever got bad back pain again, I must say that I would unhesitatingly seek the advice of my local physiotherapists.

Summing up

There are lots of different types of physiotherapy. The scientific evidence in favour of some of them is a little lacking, but it does seem to be undisputed that physiotherapeutic treatment that involves exercise, and getting you moving, should help speed your recovery.

Physiotherapy isn't likely to *cure* your backache on its own. However, large numbers of those with back pain report that after seeing a physiotherapist, and being shown how to adjust their lifestyles, they feel a lot better and have less pain.

9

Long-term (chronic) backache

I said at the beginning of this book that most people who develop backache will get better fairly quickly. Unfortunately, though, that isn't so for *everybody*.

Quite a few men and women experience back pain that drags on and on, lasting months or even years. It's for such people that this particular chapter is intended. If you've had back pain for, say, six months or more, and things don't seem to be improving, then please read the advice I'm about to give.

However, in this section I'm *not* talking about 'root pain' (usually caused by a disc problem). That's dealt with in Chapter 10.

Chronic backache

People often think that the word 'chronic' means 'very severe', but that's not the case. It just means 'long-lasting'. Unfortunately, some of us do get chronic pain in the back. I know what it feels like, because at one time I had backache that went on for several years. Thank heavens, I'm free of it now.

So I can assure you: the fact that you've got chronic backache doesn't necessarily mean that you're going to have it for life. However, it can be quite miserable while it lasts.

If the pain just won't go away, this really can have a very bad effect on your life. If you have to put up with backache day after day, that can make you feel pretty down in the dumps. And if you're always stiff and limited in your movements, that may make you feel old and 'past it'. It's easy to become really fed up, or even clinically depressed.

Sadly, I have quite often seen people with chronic back pain who've run into trouble with their:

- jobs;
- sex lives;
- marriages.

However, chronic backache doesn't *have* to ruin these areas of your life. Let's consider them in turn.

Chronic backache and your job

We'll look first at the question of jobs. If you're in the building trade, or have some other employment that involves heavy lifting, then it's easy to see that chronic backache could mean that you can't work – or that you become so inefficient that you get the sack.

But even people who are in 'non-lifting' jobs can find themselves out of work because of back pain. After all, if you are in such discomfort that you find difficulty in getting to work in the morning, and are always late, or have trouble sitting at your desk, or (quite importantly) you keep on and on complaining about your back … then, alas, you become a much less attractive employment prospect.

Indeed, a lot of folk get 'signed off' by their doctors as unable to work because of 'back trouble' or a 'back strain', and continue collecting certificates and drawing sick pay or incapacity benefit for years on end. (Whether this will change, as a result of the government's controversial scheme to get people off incapacity benefit, remains to be seen.)

However, as we'll see in a moment, many people with backache *can* return to some form of work – and it can sometimes be quite good for their backs.

Take the case of one of my patients, Harry. He was a plumber – a trade that is notoriously associated with 'bad backs', because it involves so much stooping and tugging, and trying to wriggle through confined spaces. When Harry developed pain in the lower back, both he and I thought he would be fit again soon.

But he wasn't. Six months later, he was still in a lot of pain, and he had lost his job.

For a while, he just sat around, drinking and smoking too much, experiencing a lot of pain, and feeling very sorry for himself.

But then he realized that, at 45, his working life *wasn't* over. He took a course in book-keeping, and within a few months he was able to open his own plumbing business, with the help of his wife. He was soon employing his two sons, who were both trained plumbers, plus a couple of guys from Poland. These days, Harry sits at a desk, with a computer and a phone.

Interestingly, from the time when he started this little business, he found that his backache was more bearable. It hadn't disappeared – but he could manage it.

That's not uncommon. People who go back to work often find that their back pain and stiffness ease up as a result of the amount of movement involved in the job. I'm not suggesting, though, that if your work involves heavy lifting, you should go back to it, come what may. There are certain types of heavy manual labour that should, in my view, be 'off limits' for people who have really bad backs.

However, lying or sitting around is the worst possible thing for chronic back pain. So even if you can't work, you can help yourself by taking daily exercise.

Chronic backache and your sex life

What about people's sex lives if they have back pain? Regrettably, it's very easy to allow backache to mess up your physical relationship with your partner. After all, if you get a pain whenever you roll over in bed, or when you thrust your hips forward, that does tend to limit your sexual activities a bit.

I have actually known middle-aged men and women who've said to me: 'Oh, I know my love life's over now, doctor. I'll never be able to manage it again.' In a few cases, I've managed to convince them that this is *not* true, and have been able to persuade them that they can resume sexual intercourse, or maybe just 'love play'. Take the case of Shane ...

At 41 years of age, he was hit by severe low backache. It didn't respond very well to treatment, and he found it particularly difficult to lie in bed. Sometimes he sat up in a chair all night. After about a year of this, he managed to convince himself that the pain was so bad that he really couldn't have intercourse again. So he gave up on sex altogether.

What he didn't know – but I *did* – was that his wife Gloria had become so frustrated that she started seeking satisfaction elsewhere, with a handsome young man at her workplace. She had come to my surgery and told me this.

In an effort to help, I pointed out to Shane that while his back problem might make it too uncomfortable to have intercourse, there was no known form of lower-back trouble that could stop a man cuddling his wife, and bringing her to a climax in other ways. I also suggested that an hour before attempting any sexual activity, he took a couple of pain-killers. Much to my relief, he accepted this advice.

As a result, this couple managed to keep their sex life going, and Gloria ended her dalliance with the young man at work. When I last saw Shane, they were getting on very well, and he reported that his back pain was slowly improving.

Chronic back pain and your marriage

It is a sad fact that some men and women who have chronic backache do run into marital difficulties, and even get divorced. This can be partly because of the sort of sexual difficulties that I've just mentioned.

Also, it's a fact that some spouses are less than happy when the lively, active person who they married becomes a semi-invalid who can't go anywhere or do anything, or even enjoy themselves. But again, this problem is *not* insuperable.

Take the case of Felicity. She and her husband used to love going ballroom dancing together, until she developed a painful back problem. Her immediate response was to give up dancing immediately. Also, she more or less refused to go out at all. So all the fun they used to have with friends vanished overnight.

Her husband Bill found that his social life had disappeared. His reaction was to start spending most of his evenings in the pub. He met an attractive dancing partner there, and guess what happened? Within a year, Felicity and Bill were divorced.

In an odd way, this had quite a beneficial effect on Felicity. She realized that her pain had made her quite phobic about going out, so she found herself a counsellor who encouraged her to get out and about, and to develop a new circle of friends. Some regular sessions with an osteopath made her less stiff and more mobile. She has a new partner. And I'm not sure that she misses Bill very much now.

Keeping moving and being positive

Where backache is concerned, there have been two big health discoveries in recent years. The first is that exercise – and not rest – is good for back pain.

Until late on in the twentieth century, people who had chronic back pain were told that they must rest, at all costs. Often, they were put in corsets – or even in appallingly restrictive, hard-plaster jackets. They were advised to spend a lot of their time lying flat. Often, they were supposed to do this on a hard board, or even on the floor.

All that has gone out of vogue now. Those with back pain are generally encouraged by their physiotherapists and other health professionals to keep moving. No one expects them to run marathons – unless they really want to – but gentle exercise is universally recognized as beneficial.

The second big discovery has been that people who have a positive attitude are more likely to get better from illness. This applies to many medical conditions – including backache.

Why that should be so isn't entirely clear, but I must say that I have seen evidence of it again and again. The man who comes into the surgery full of woe is generally slow to recover from back pain. The woman who walks in, clearly full of determination to defeat her back problem, probably *will* beat it.

Some authorities on the subject say that if you blame your job and your boss for your back pain, then your anger will help to prevent you from recovering. I have not been able to find scientific proof of this. However, I have seen cases where people who are pursuing legal compensation for back pain make absolutely no progress – until they get a cash settlement. *Then* they start making progress ...

This doesn't necessarily mean that they have been malingering. I think it just shows the power of the human mind over the body – even in cases of backache.

Chronic backache and helping yourself

So if you have chronic backache, it's very important to be positive – and to make every effort to help yourself. Unfortunately, pills from a doctor aren't likely to cure you.

But things that can help you recover are:

- getting fitter;
- losing weight – if you're carrying too many pounds;
- giving up smoking (it has recently been shown that smoking is bad for the blood supply of the back);
- taking daily exercise.

Also, you really *must* avoid the things that so often make backache worse. If you've read the early part of this book, you'll know that these are:

- lifting in unsafe ways;
- bending;
- twisting – especially in cars;
- sitting with poor posture and with your spine badly supported.

Don't give up on professional help

If you have chronic back pain, it's easy to start thinking that 'nothing can be done'. Some people stop going to their doctor's – except to pick up prescriptions for pain-killers (see below).

Others give up on their physiotherapist, osteopath or chiropractor. Personally, I don't think this is a good idea, though where the therapy is private, it's understandable that those who are short of cash may not feel able to keep on paying out.

However, do please try and keep in touch with your GP, physiotherapist or other health professional. It's good to have them assessing your condition regularly – and there is always the chance that they may come up with some brand-new idea to help you.

Avoid strong pain-killers

Unfortunately, there is quite a tendency among people with chronic back pain to get 'hooked' on pain-killing drugs. This is very easily done if you are constantly in pain. No matter how strong-minded you are, though, you can become habituated to these pills.

And I'm sorry to say that there are a few GPs who just keep issuing prescriptions for strong pain-killing drugs, without really thinking about the consequences. In particular, there is a medication called 'tramadol' (trade names Zamadol and Zydol) that in recent years has been far too commonly dished out for long-term back pain.

Related to morphia, tramadol can cause sedation, tiredness, tummy upsets, fainting and many other side-effects. Most importantly, it affects the *mind* – often making you feel woozy and muddled. It interacts with alcohol – tending to increase the degree of intoxication – and with various other drugs.

Not surprisingly, there is a ready market for it among drug addicts, some of whom will enthusiastically steal prescriptions for tramadol, and indeed sell tramadol capsules to one another. This is *not* a drug that you want to be taking long term.

Full information about drugs for back pain is given in Chapter 5.

Getting emotional/psychological help

If the pain is really getting you down, please don't be embarrassed to seek psychological help. In fact, if you're clinically depressed, then you should definitely see your GP to talk things over.

She may well suggest putting you on anti-depressants. Although the value of these drugs has recently been questioned, they do seem to help quite a few people to cope with debilitating pain.

Also, if somebody's life is being made really miserable by any illness – including back disorders – there is quite a chance that counselling or psychotherapy could help. In particular, please consider cognitive behavioural therapy (CBT), which has become very popular recently. In essence, it's a way of helping people to *think differently* about their problems.

I have seen cases in which it helped people who were in pain to alter their way of thinking so that the pain was still there, but was no longer 'first and foremost' in their minds. That was a change that was well worth having.

It's worth trying new things

The important thing is not to give up hope. Some people do get a spontaneous improvement in their chronic pain. And, however long your backache goes on, it's worth being on the look-out for new things that might help. Innovative treatments do come along, and there's always the chance that your doctor, physiotherapist or chiropractor/osteopath may come up with something fresh that would help you.

Please keep an open mind, and don't say 'Oh, there's *nothing* that would do me any good.' There may be *something*.

In particular, I think that anyone with chronic back pain should take a look at Chapter 11, which lists the common alternative treatments used in cases of backache. Among them, I'd specially like to draw your attention to the famous 'Alexander technique'. It genuinely does re-adjust and stretch the spine, and I have seen it help people who have had backache for many years.

The 'back swing' and other traction devices

Those with chronic back pain may perhaps benefit from various commercially produced traction (i.e. stretching) devices. They are pretty expensive – ranging from £179 to £1,165 – so I don't feel you should rush into buying one. My suggestion: take the advice of a physiotherapist first, and perhaps let her try out traction on you in her clinic/department. Only if she thinks that one of these devices would help, should you go ahead and purchase – unless, of course, money is no object to you!

These inventions all work by the principle of 'inversion therapy'. This means that they turn you upside down, so that your own body weight puts traction on your spine. For years, the best-known one was the 'back swing'. I demonstrated this device several times on television, and I always found it pleasant and soothing to hang from – though it did make reading the autocue a little difficult.

These days, there are numerous other inversion machines, including the Infinity Inversion Table, and also various models of the Teeter. More details are available from <www.naturalliving.co.uk>.

The hanging upside-down boots

These boots were invented by a Californian physician, and have proved very popular in the USA. I visited the doctor in Pasadena for a demonstration, and found that they are rather like mountain boots with big hooks on the front – so that you can hang upside-down from a stout metal rail. Once again, the idea is to stretch your spine.

I must add that although I found the boots fun to use, it was clear that you need to be pretty athletic in order to hang yourself head-down like a bat, from a rail positioned two metres off the ground.

Also, if anything went wrong, there would be a very nasty crash.

TENS machines

Rather more practical for most people with chronic back pain is the TENS machine, which I mentioned briefly earlier in the book. These are useful little pain-relieving devices, and nowadays many of those with backache buy or hire them, in order to ease the pain. But they don't work for everyone.

The letters 'TENS' stand for 'Transcutaneous Electrical Nerve Stimulation'. The machine delivers small electrical pulses to your body, through electrodes placed on your skin. For reasons that are still not totally clear, these pulses seem to do two things:

1 They help to block a 'pain pathway' to your brain.
2 They probably stimulate your body to produce its own natural pain-killers (endorphins).

Sometimes you can borrow a TENS machine on the NHS, particularly if you're attending a physiotherapy clinic. But, these days, most people buy them – partly because there are big ads for them in the national papers. Currently, the cost is between £14.50 and £65.

(*Note*: Please do not use a TENS machine if you're pregnant, or have epilepsy, or use a cardiac pacemaker.)

The new 'IDD' method

Since early 2008, there has been a great deal of advertising in the UK press, and on the internet, for something called 'IDD therapy'. Its marketing slogan is: 'Puts back pain behind you'.

IDD stands for 'Intervertebral Differential Dynamics'. This is described as 'an advanced, computer-controlled physiotherapy programme for long-term back relief'. It is claimed that some 100,000 people have been treated since 2001.

The general idea is that computerized technology is used in order to target 'selected vertebrae', and that is done by using something called 'the Accu-SPINA spinal care device'. This device is said to apply 'distraction' – which, it is claimed, creates a negative pressure in your discs.

The advertising literature states that 'secondary oscillating waveforms target the supporting soft tissues surrounding the injured site, releasing spasmodic behaviour and crucially increasing strength and flexibility'. Apparently, all this can be done without taking your clothes off.

The general plan is that you have 20 treatments lasting 25 to 30 minutes each, spread over a six-week period. This will certainly be quite expensive, particularly as you will need to have an MRI scan. An initial consultation with the IDD company's orthopaedic consultant currently costs £125, though reductions are possible. After his preliminary assessment, your treatment is supervised by a physiotherapist.

I must stress that I myself haven't tried IDD, but I hope that it will turn out to be as good as its literature claims. If you want to know more, look at the website <www.iddtherapy.co.uk>.

For completeness, I should add that there has been some adverse comment about IDD on the internet. I have no idea who is right in this matter.

Summing up

Having long-lasting backache is no fun. But some people do get better spontaneously; others find ways of coping. And there is always the chance that some new treatment will come along.

Please be guided by your health professional. And whatever you do, don't give up!

10

Nerve root pain – and the famous disc

In this chapter, we'll deal with disc trouble and how it causes back pain by pressing on the nerve roots. But let me point out that 'slipped discs' (also known as 'herniated' or 'prolapsed' discs) only make up a small proportion of cases of backache – in fact, probably less than 5 per cent.

So if you have back pain, but haven't got a prolapsed disc, then please don't bother with this chapter. It doesn't apply to you.

What is nerve root pain?

In this book, I've several times mentioned 'nerve root pain'. This is pain that occurs because something is pressing on the roots of the nerves, just where they emerge from your spinal cord.

In the great majority of cases, what presses on the nerve roots is a bulging *disc*. There are other possible culprits, such as a collapsed vertebra, but these are uncommon.

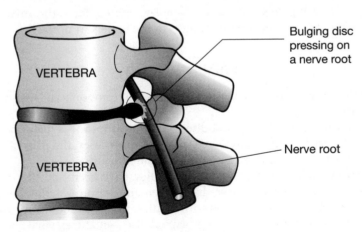

Figure 10.1 Disc causing nerve root pain

You can see the nerve roots of the lower part of the back in Figure 10.1. You will also notice that something is poking out from between the bones of the spine (the vertebrae) and is pressing against one of the roots. That 'something' is a bulging or 'slipped' disc.

What is a slipped disc?

In Chapter 2, I mentioned that a disc is like a tiny, greyish burger, made out of cartilage. It acts as a shock absorber in the spine. But unfortunately, as a result of stresses on the back, it can bulge out ('prolapse' or 'herniate') from between the bones – a bit like a blob of putty squeezing out from between your fingers.

That bulge may produce no symptoms. But if the disc presses on your nerve roots, then you will probably experience great pain. *And you will feel that pain in the area supplied by the nerve root.*

Disc trouble can happen in any part of the back. But far and away the most common site is the lumbar region – that is, the area just above your buttocks. This is because the lumbar discs and vertebrae are subjected to more strain than anywhere else, as we bend, lift and twist around.

So the nerve roots that are most frequently affected by pressure from a bulging disc are the ones emerging from the lower part of your lumbar spine. And those nerve roots come together to form the *sciatic nerve*, which supplies the back of your leg.

Therefore, the most likely results of a prolapsed disc are:

- pain in the lumbar region – usually located just above one buttock;
- pain running down the back of one leg, often as far as the ankle;
- frequently, tingling and numbness in the same part of the leg.

What is sciatica?

Nearly everyone has heard the word 'sciatica' (pronounced 'sigh-ATT-ee-ka').

A lot of people think it's a disease, but all it means is 'pain in the region served by the sciatic nerve'. And in most cases, the pain of sciatica is caused by one of those troublesome little discs.

Rather oddly, some people say that they have been told that they have sciatica – but have never been given any reason *why* they've got it. So if you've been diagnosed with sciatica, then you should ask your doctor whether it's caused by a prolapsed disc – and, if so, what can be done about it.

Diagnosing a disc problem

Generally speaking, the diagnosis of disc trouble isn't too difficult. Your doctor, osteopath, chiropractor or physiotherapist will be able to make a pretty good guess at the diagnosis if you say that you've got lumbar pain that runs down the back of your leg towards your heel.

Any of these health professionals should be expert in examining you, to check out precisely where you are feeling the pain. They may also check to see if there is any impairment of sensation (i.e. feeling) in your leg, and whether your leg reflexes have been affected.

They will certainly do the well-known Straight Leg Raising (SLR) test. In this, the examiner gets you to lie flat, then tries to lift your leg while supporting it under the ankle.

In fit, healthy people, it should be possible to lift the leg to an upright position. But when a disc is pressing on the roots of the sciatic nerve, then the amount of elevation will be sharply limited by the pain that the person feels.

What about X-rays? Contrary to what a lot of people think, X-rays are of very little value in diagnosing disc trouble. Alas, the discs are made of gristly material that doesn't show up on X-ray plates.

However, more specialized (and much more expensive) imaging – such as an MRI scan – may be done later on, particularly if there has to be a decision about whether you need surgery. An MRI, also known as an NMR, really *does* show up the discs.

Initial treatment of a disc problem

The good news about 'slipped discs' is that a lot of them get better within about six weeks. So, in the early stages, it's likely that everyone will want to treat you 'conservatively' – in other words, they won't want to suggest early surgery, except perhaps if you live in the USA.

Why does the disc problem get better on its own? That's quite a difficult question to answer, because we can't actually *look* at it as it improves. However, it's probable that the bulge gradually 'shrinks down' or even withers away. In some cases, the disc may actually go back into its normal place, which is located entirely between two vertebrae – with no bits sticking out.

Anyway, it is virtually certain that during those first six weeks or so, your doctor will *not* want you to go in for any kind of dramatic treatment. She will suggest:

- rest;
- gentle exercise;

- pain-killers;
- anti-inflammatories;
- warmth to the affected area;
- avoiding lifting, bending and twisting.

If you decide to go to chiropractors or osteopaths, they will certainly try manipulative techniques on your lumbar spine. Do these make the disc 'go back'?

That's extremely hard to say, but some do report that 'there was a click, and everything was OK'. And a lot of folk are definitely improved by the manipulations, and come away feeling less pain.

In my own case, when I had bad disc trouble I went to a succession of osteopaths and chiropractors. They tried very hard, but were unable to make my disc go back into place.

But, in fairness to them, they did nearly always ease my discomfort and stiffness.

More specialized treatments for disc problems

If your nerve root pain isn't starting to improve after about six weeks, you should start thinking about getting some different kind of treatment. Possibilities include:

- physiotherapy (see Chapter 8), and particularly exercises and Cyriax or Maitland manipulation;
- epidural injections – which are very similar to the pain-killing ones used in childbirth; they often produce instant relief from pain, but unfortunately this may only last a short time;
- nerve root injections (rare);
- osteopathy or chiropractic – if you haven't already tried them;
- sclerosant therapy: a method no longer much used in the UK, which involves injecting 'hardening' fluid near the disc.

Surgery

In the UK and many other countries, surgery tends to be a bit of a 'last resort' for disc problems. This isn't so in the USA, where disc operations are far more common.

But wherever you live, there may come a time when the efforts of your health professionals clearly aren't paying off, and you decide that you must ask a surgeon to see what he can do.

Please bear in mind that although the results of surgery are often brilliant, not all operations are successful. And, invariably, you will need to work hard afterwards, with the aid of the physiotherapists, to get the best results.

All surgical procedures for 'slipped discs' have the same objective: to relieve the pressure on the nerve roots. Your surgeon, or one of his staff, should explain clearly to you what they plan to do. But here are the most usual operations for curing a bulging disc:

- *Laminectomy* (*Decompression*). This is the traditional operation for disc trouble. As you lie flat on your face, your surgeon makes a vertical incision in the small of your back. Through it, he removes all or part of the troublesome disc. The operation is called 'laminectomy' because part of a vertebra is called the 'lamina', and the surgeon has to remove that bit in order to get at your disc.
- *Microdiscectomy*. This is a modern and 'milder' version of the above. A small amount of bone is removed, together with the bulging disc material underneath it.
- *DIAM insertion*. This is not so common. The letters 'DIAM' stand for 'Device for Intervertebral Assisted Motion'. This means that the surgeon inserts an H-shaped implant between two vertebrae, in order to take the pressure off the nerve root.
- *Disc nucleus replacement*. This means putting an artificial 'centre' into the middle of a damaged disc. Unlike most other spinal 'ops', this one is usually done from the front.
- *Total disc replacement*. This means what it says: replacing the whole battered disc with an artificial one, usually made of metal.
- *Fusion*. This is an operation in which the surgeon fuses (i.e. fixes) two or more bones of the spine together, so as to prevent movement and therefore reduce pain. It is used in degenerative disc disease, and also to treat some fractures, and in cases where the back is abnormally curved. The operation involves 'splinting' two vertebrae together by using either a bone graft taken from elsewhere in the body, or else a synthetic bone substitute. Rods and screws are generally needed in order to hold these in place. Your spine may be a little stiffer after a bone fusion, but there should generally be a lot less pain.

Summing up

It's a bit alarming to be told that you've got a protruding disc, but in a lot of cases the problem will clear up within six weeks. If it doesn't, there are many treatments that can help.

In the UK and most other countries, only a minority of people who have disc trouble will need surgery. However, the results of an operation by a surgeon who specializes in this field are usually very good.

11

Alternative strategies for back pain

Many people turn to alternative medicine for help with their backache, particularly when it's been going on for a long time. If you have
chronic back pain, it's very likely that someone will suggest to you that
an alternative technique might help you.

So in this chapter, I list 32 of the most commonly employed types
of 'complementary' therapy, together with a very brief description. This
may help you to decide whether the treatments would appeal to you or
not.

As a doctor, I am of course trained to look for scientific evidence that
might prove the usefulness of any form of treatment. Unfortunately, as
we've seen in earlier chapters, it's quite difficult to prove scientifically
that anything *definitely* works in cases of backache.

So in this chapter, I've simply tried to tell you what the 'alternatives'
are, and to avoid letting my own opinion of them obtrude.

However, in a couple of cases (notably the Alexander technique), the
relevance of the treatment to your bad back is pretty obvious – and in
these instances, I have abandoned my impartiality and said 'This one
is worth trying.'

In contrast, as regards one or two other types of therapy, if the arguments for them seem quite bizarre to me, I've said so. However, one
must never discount the famous 'placebo effect'. For the plain fact is
that if you give human beings *any* treatment – no matter how crazy – it
will work for some of them, at least for a while.

Placebos can lower your blood pressure, make you lose weight, or
cure your headaches – though sometimes only temporarily. If you
believe in them, they will do you good for a time. And if your doctor
or therapist tells you that *he* believes passionately in them, the effect
on you is likely to be even greater.

So here is the list. Some of these therapies may well operate by the
mysterious power of suggestion, but if they help relieve your back pain,
that can only be good.

Acupressure

This is a system that may well relieve pain. It is very similar to acupuncture (see below), but uses pressure with the fingertips instead of needles. Acupressure is related to shiatsu.

Acupuncture

Acupuncture is a system of therapy that involves placing needles at various points in the skin, in accordance with the 'meridians' laid down by traditional Chinese medicine.

Acupuncture is of course used throughout the world these days. Western doctors do now generally accept that it is effective in relieving pain, including backache. It is widely employed in the UK at NHS pain clinics. At a conference in Hong Kong, I saw some evidence that it increases the flow of endorphins, which are the body's natural pain-killers.

However, it is hard to see how acupuncture could possibly *correct* mechanical problems in the back. Nevertheless, I think it's often worth a try.

Contrary to what many people fear, the needles don't cause pain. However, *electrical* acupuncture – in which a current is passed through the needles – can be extremely painful if the dial has been wrongly set! This happened to me once in Kowloon.

Alexander technique

This is well worth trying if you have a long-term back problem. Frederick Matthias Alexander (1865–1955), a Tasmanian actor, was what the Australians call a 'larrikin' – in other words, a bit of a rogue. However, he did spot that many of us have very poor posture, and that our spines tend to be out of true. He then came up with a brilliant system for improving the positioning of the skeleton, and particularly the spinal bones.

One simple Alexander manoeuvre is to pretend that you have a cord attached to the top of your skull, and that it is drawing you upwards and making you taller. This stretches out your spine. Indeed, if you undergo Alexander training, you probably *will* get marginally taller.

The Alexander technique received an enormous boost in August 2008, when the *British Medical Journal* published a paper originating from the Universities of Bristol and Southampton. The researchers looked at over 500 people who had recurrent back pain. They were put on various regimes, including massage and the Alexander technique.

This well-organized trial revealed that massage was initially good at relieving pain, though the benefits didn't last. However, those who were given 'Alexander lessons' reported lessened pain and greater mobility – and these benefits lasted for at least a year.

If you want to try 'Alexander', you should consult one of the many teachers of the Alexander technique that can be found via the internet, or in *Yellow Pages*. Sessions tend to cost around £30 a time, and you will probably need a number of them. But bear in mind that the *British Medical Journal* trial showed that just *six* lessons were of almost as much value as 24.

It would also be worth looking at Dr Wilfred Barlow's excellent books *The Alexander Principle* and *More Talk of Alexander*. And you can check out the website of the Society of Teachers of the Alexander Technique at: <www.stat.org.uk>.

Aromatherapy

Most people find aromatherapy a pleasant form of alternative medicine, in which agreeable-smelling essential oils and other plant extracts are used in order to induce relaxation and to try to relieve pain. These agents can be applied to the skin, inhaled, or mixed into warm baths. The brave sometimes take them rectally or even vaginally (not to be done unless recommended by a *qualified* aromatherapist).

Autogenics

This is a relaxation-inducing technique, involving a series of attention-focusing mental exercises. It is claimed that it helps self-healing. Autogenics was particularly popular in the 1990s.

Ayurvedic medicine

Ayurvedic medicine is the term applied to a huge, complex and ancient system that originates with the *Vedas* – a large body of sacred Hindu texts, written well before the Christian era. They give a lot of good medical advice, but inevitably much of what they say is not very relevant to today's world.

There are countless ayurvedic practitioners in Asia, and their influence has spread to the West in recent decades. They don't all speak with one voice, so there is no single ayurvedic teaching. Much of their therapy depends on herbs (particularly herbs collected in India), meditation and massage.

In 2004, the *Journal of the American Medical Association* reported that some ayurvedic pills contained unacceptable levels of heavy metals. I once sat on a General Medical Council case in which it was revealed that certain ayurvedic preparations contained faecal bacteria.

So, if you choose ayurvedic medicine to treat your backache, take care that you are getting your medication from a reputable supplier.

Bach remedies

This is a system of treatment based on dilutions of flower material in a 50:50 solution of water and brandy. The remedies are widely believed to promote relaxation and improve mood. As Dr Bach's family originated in Wales, the name should be pronounced in the Welsh fashion, rather than as 'batch'.

Its usefulness in back pain must surely be limited, but you might find it soothing.

Bowen

This is a remedial technique that has increased in popularity in recent years. It's a hands-on method in which the fingers and thumbs are employed to make gentle, rolling movements, thereby producing calmness and aiming to relieve pain.

Chinese herbalism

Herbal medicine has a long and honourable history, in India, China and elsewhere. Devotees of Chinese herbalism claim that it will relieve back pain. However, it seems unlikely that the herbs could actually alter mechanical derangements in your spine – though maybe it could ease pain.

Unfortunately, in recent years, it's become clear that some herbal products sold in the West may contain dangerous levels of mercury and arsenic. A few even contain steroids – which might account for their effectiveness in rheumatic disorders.

Also, some Chinese herbal medications sold in the UK have been found to contain the herb aristolochia, which can cause kidney disease.

So, it is clear you need to take care and buy only from a reputable supplier or qualified herbalist.

Colour therapy

It is claimed that the wavelengths of certain colours can be matched with the wavelength emitted by certain diseases. Thus, say practitioners, if you could find a colour that 'matches' your spinal problem, that would be helpful. Likely? I think not.

Colonic irrigation/colonic hydrotherapy

This means introducing a liquid, such as warm water, into the rectum, via a tube inserted through the anus. The contents of the bowel (i.e. faeces) are then washed out. The idea is to remove toxins, and therefore help all kinds of symptoms, including back pain.

This type of treatment sprang into popularity in European spa centres during the nineteenth century. At an Italian spa a few years ago, I was offered colonic therapy with a jet of natural mineral water, in order to relieve my backache. Murmuring *'Non, grazie; io sono britannico,'* I politely declined.

Deep tissue massage

This is one of the many different types of massage that are available these days. Deep tissue massage tends to be carried out in gyms and leisure centres. It is described as 'holistic and restorative', producing profound relaxation.

Practitioners say that it is good for back pain, and various other symptoms related to joints and the musculo-skeletal system. Its aim seems to be to penetrate deeply into your muscles, and muscle stretches are often part of the package.

On logical grounds, it does seem likely that deep tissue massage could help ease backache and back stiffness. Costs are often quite high – for instance, £105 for a series of three massages.

Herbalism

People have been using herbal therapy for thousands of years, and today there seems to be renewed interest in this type of treatment. It is often claimed that it will help backache. However, there are no scientific studies to support this.

Among the main varieties of herbal medicine are Chinese (see above) and Indian types – the latter including ayurvedic (see above) and Unani herbalism. In Britain, it may be a good idea to go to a practitioner who belongs to the National Institute of Medical Herbalists, whose website is: <www.nimh.org.uk>.

Homeopathy

This is a system of medicine based on the idea that disorders can be treated with agents that produce similar symptoms to those of the disease, provided they are diluted enough.

Orthodox doctors claim that in fact the dilution of homeopathic medicines is so enormous that there is nothing left in the medication at all. As a result, the British medical profession has tended to take a fairly benign view of homeopathy, feeling that at least it can't possibly cause any side-effects. Homeopathy's popularity has been greatly helped by the fact that it's been patronized by the royal family.

For backache, homeopaths generally recommend treatment with agents such as arnica, bryonia and aesculus. If you need homeopathic treatment, there are practitioners in virtually every large town in the UK. It is probably wise to choose one who belongs to a major professional organization, such as the Society of Homeopaths, whose website is: <www.homeopathy-soh.org>.

A very small number of GPs practise it. And you may be surprised to hear that there are still five NHS homeopathic hospitals, notably the Royal London Homeopathic – though their continued existence is looking a bit doubtful.

Hypnotherapy

Hypnotherapy is an extremely effective way of producing relaxation and relieving tensions. But, apart from its soothing and stress-relieving properties, it is hard to see that it can do a lot for backache.

Indian head massage

Also known as 'champissage', this technique has become increasingly popular since the 1970s. The idea is to 'unblock' energy flows, thus relieving pain.

Iridology

This is a system in which someone looks into your eyes, and by checking the colours in your iris aims to diagnose exactly what is wrong with your back or any other part of your body.

It is only claimed to be a method of diagnosis, not a treatment.

Kinesiology, applied

Applied kinesiology (AK) is a system of assessing muscle strength, in the back and elsewhere, by using the hand. It was invented by a chiropractor in 1964. Adherents believe that every malfunction of an organ is accompanied by a corresponding muscle dysfunction. This does not really seem very likely.

Massage

Any type of gentle massage is likely to give some relief to your backache, whether it is administered by a partner, a friend, or a professional. This is because massaging relaxes the back muscles, so that they come out of the uncomfortable spasm that so often accompanies back pain.

In the last few years, 'sports massage' has become extremely popular, particularly in gyms, hotels and leisure clubs. This term could mean anything, but a good sports masseur is probably going to administer something approximating to a 'Deep tissue massage' (see p. 102).

Meditation

There is no way that meditation can correct a mechanical derangement in your back. However, I have no doubt at all that meditation can help a lot of people who have long-term backache.

It can induce peace and relaxation, and possibly alter the perception of pain. However, you should be aware of the fact that there are many different schools of meditation. Be wary of any that want to relieve you of a lot of cash.

Transcendental meditation ('TM') is a trademarked term that refers to a form of deep meditation invented by Maharishi Mahash Yogi (of Beatles fame) back in 1958. In the UK, it has been strongly associated with the Natural Law Party.

Naturopathy

Naturopathy is a system of treatment based on the idea that the body has the inherent ability to heal itself. In the UK, naturopathy is now regulated by a General Council, and there is a register of trained naturopaths.

Nutritional therapy

It is not unreasonable to say that your health – including the health of your back – is to some extent dependent on what you eat. Nutritional therapists go further than this, and try to help you rid your body of toxic chemicals, in an effort to produce physical repair in your back and elsewhere.

Nutrition therapists prescribe varying kinds of diet and herbs, plus mineral and vitamin supplements.

Pilates

Pilates (pronounced 'pie-LAH-tees') has become massively popular in recent years – particularly among people who have long-term backache. It is a method of strengthening the postural muscles of the body, including those of the back, and developing correct alignment.

It was invented during the First World War by a German doctor called Josef Pilates who had been interned in Britain. He later developed his philosophy while working with dancers in New York and treating their injuries.

I have seen quite a few people with back pain who have found pilates helpful. It does seem to improve the 'core strength' of the back – see Chapter 13.

Radionics

I cannot in all conscience recommend radionics to those with back pain, though it is certainly free of side-effects. In a nutshell, it is a system that is dependent on the idea that a disordered part of your body, such as your back, can radiate an abnormal wave form, and that this wave form can be recognized by a practitioner at a distance.

A variant of this idea is the famous 'black box' diagnostic apparatus. The idea is that the radionics practitioner can place a sample of your hair or blood in a box that contains various electrical coils. He then uses the box to diagnose the exact cause of your problem, and recommends appropriate treatment.

My views of radionics are admittedly coloured by the fact that years ago I sent a sample of hair to a black-box practitioner, who diagnosed that I had all sorts of unlikely illnesses. In fact, the hairs came from my cat Sooty!

Reflexology

Another popular system of treatment; in reflexology the practitioner massages the subject's feet – and occasionally her hands as well. The idea is that on the soles of the feet there are 'reflex areas' that correspond to various parts of the body. One particular area is supposed to represent the back.

Most devotees appear to believe that this pressure on the soles of the feet can unlock 'energy channels'.

Reiki

This is pronounced as 'ray-key', and is a Japanese system of treatment in which the person lies on a couch, and the practitioner holds her hands out over him in various positions. The belief is that energy is being moved through the palms. Full sessions take an hour or so.

Rolfing

Rolfing is a hands-on connective tissue manipulation, which aims to relieve stress and pain. It is named after its founder, Ida Rolf. The name 'Rolfing' is a registered trade mark.

Shiatsu

This is a Japanese system of massage. The word 'shiatsu' actually means 'finger pressure'. Essentially, this is a form of acupressure (see above), which aims to relieve pain through exploiting the meridians of acupuncture.

Swedish massage

The Swedes, with their long traditions of sport, gymnastics and fitness, have always been keen advocates of massage. Their variety of it has spread throughout the Western world. It falls into five categories: petrissage, tapotement, effleurage, friction and vibration.

It will certainly ease muscle spasm in your back, and may relieve pain and stiffness to some degree.

Tai chi ch'uan

Usually abbreviated to tai chi, 'Tai chi ch'uan' means in English something approximating to 'Great clunking fist'. While there is indeed a martial arts aspect to tai chi, it is also a philosophical discipline.

But furthermore, the term applies to the 'health exercises' that people can be seen doing in public parks all over China.

These graceful, balletic movements seem to make people feel better, and increase their strength and suppleness. It is also sometimes claimed to help in various illnesses, including musculo-skeletal aches and pains.

While the scientific evidence for that is lacking, common sense suggests that this gentle rhythmic stretching would probably be worth trying if you have a long-term back problem.

Unani

Unani is a system of treatment said to have begun in ancient Greece, and to have eventually been taken to South Asia by the Mogul conquerors.

It is largely dependent on herbal therapy, and is still very popular in India, especially in Muslim communities.

Yoga

A lot of people with long-term back pain decide to give yoga a try, and some of them report that they benefit from it. As I'm sure you know, yoga is a very ancient Indian discipline which aims for harmony of mind, body and spirit.

There are many different types of yoga, including hatha, astanga, bikram and sivananda. They all seem to have the capacity to induce serenity and relaxation, which is quite useful if you are being plagued by back pain.

Yoga also appears to improve muscle tone and posture – and perhaps core strength (see Chapter 13). Obviously, you should not get into any yoga position that produces pain in your back.

12

Serious – but uncommon – causes of backache

I need to emphasize that most really serious causes of back pain are quite rare. So if you've just got what your doctor, physiotherapist or osteopath says is perfectly 'ordinary' backache, then I don't think you should waste your time – and cause yourself alarm – by reading this chapter.

In Chapter 5, I listed a number of symptoms that could indicate that a pain in your back might be due to something serious. All up-to-date health professionals know these 'Red Flag' symptoms. Indeed, if you ever ring up the 'Dial-a-Physiotherapist' service mentioned in Chapter 8, the physiotherapist's first concern would be to ensure that you don't have any such warning features.

But say you *do* have some 'Red Flag' symptoms, then what are the serious illnesses that they might suggest? I'll deal with these alphabetically:

Ankylosing spondylitis

Ankylosing spondylitis (AS) – also known as 'bamboo spine' – occurs mainly in men. It usually starts causing trouble in the 15–27 age group. Persistent backache is rare in this age range, so continuing pain in the lower back in a young man is in itself a 'Red Flag' symptom.

Approximately 1 in 900 males get AS. The early features are pain and stiffness, particularly in the lumbar region, and especially in the mornings. X-rays show that the lower vertebrae have become fused together ('ankylosed'). The sacro-iliac (S-I) joints are also affected. Most of those diagnosed with AS have a blood antigen called HLA B27, which is uncommon in the rest of the population. Other blood tests will suggest that inflammation is going on.

The cause of AS isn't known, but there are theories that it might be started off by infection. Once the diagnosis is made, it's essential that you put yourself in the care of a consultant rheumatologist, who will prescribe drug treatment, exercises and physiotherapy. The once-popular use of radiotherapy to the spine has now been abandoned as too dangerous.

Cauda equina syndrome

This is a medical emergency. Its rather odd name comes from the fact that the 'sheaf' of nerve roots in the very lowest part of the back look rather like the tail of a horse. Doctors – with their penchant for half-remembered bits of classical learning – therefore christened it with the Latin phrase for 'horsey tail'.

What happens in cauda equina syndrome (CES) is that something presses on this bundle of nerve roots. The results are likely to be:

- pain in the lower back;
- pain down one or both legs;
- loss of sensation (feeling) in the crotch area;
- bladder problems;
- bowel problems;
- loss of sexual sensation;
- sometimes, paralysis in the legs.

Frequently, the 'culprit' that is pressing on the roots is a prolapsed disc (see Chapter 10). Other causes include massive physical injury and spinal stenosis (see below). It is imperative that the person is seen by a surgeon – preferably a neurosurgeon – as quickly as possible. He may well operate to relieve the compression.

A useful website for those with long-term CES is: <www.oldcity.org.uk/cauda_equina>.

Infections in the spine

These are so rare that I think I have seen less than five cases in my life. The person develops unexplained back pain, usually accompanied by a fever. Treatment depends on the nature of the infection, but will probably include antibiotics.

Osteomalacia

People often confuse osteomalacia with osteoporosis (see below). Osteomalacia is much more rare than osteoporosis. It is a softening of bones, caused by various factors such as lack of calcium in the diet, lack of vitamin D (due to lack of sunlight), and sometimes intestinal problems – which prevent the absorption of nutrients.

The chief symptoms are bone pain and muscle weakness. Treatment is with vitamin D and calcium.

Osteoporosis

Maybe I shouldn't really have put osteoporosis in the 'uncommon causes of backache' chapter, because the fact is that it *is* very common in older people (especially women), and it can sometimes cause backache.

Osteoporosis is the famous 'thin bone' or 'fragile bone' condition, which affects many people after the age of about 55 or 60. Because the bones are so thin and therefore brittle, they are very likely to break. The common sites for these fractures are the wrist and the hip, but they can occur in the vertebrae. You may well have noticed that many old people walk around stooped forwards, as if they were looking at the ground. This 'hump-backed' appearance is due to collapse of the fronts of the vertebrae, caused by the thinness of the bone structure.

The reason why more women than men get osteoporosis is the fact that after the menopause, they lose the protective effect of their female hormones.

In an ideal world, we would be able to prevent osteoporosis completely. Good preventative measures include:

- getting lots of exercise throughout life;
- avoiding, at all costs, sitting around doing nothing;
- avoiding excessive alcohol;
- avoiding smoking.

Unfortunately, at the moment we are *not* preventing it, as evidenced by the fact that 40 per cent of women aged 65-plus will get a fracture in the wrist or elsewhere. So if you're a senior citizen and you develop a persistent pain in your back – maybe accompanied by the forward bending known as a 'dowager's hump' – ask your GP if it could perhaps be osteoporosis.

The diagnosis can be made by various specialized tests, the most common of which is a type of low-dose X-ray called a 'DEXA-scan'.

Treatment of osteoporosis is outside the scope of this book, but may involve taking calcium and vitamin D supplements, drugs called 'bisphosphonates', possibly hormones, and perhaps drugs from a group called 'SERMS'. These mimic the action of the female hormone oestrogen; the best-known SERM is raloxifene (Evista). You should also take care to get plenty of exercise.

Much more information is available from the National Osteoporosis Society, at: <www.nos.org.uk>.

Spinal stenosis

There is a tunnel (the spinal canal) that runs vertically through the vertebrae, and at its lower end it is not very wide – say, about half an inch (1.2 cm) across. Nerve roots run through this confined part of the tunnel.

'Stenosis' means narrowing. In this case, it means narrowing of that confined part of the spinal canal. The constriction can press on the nerve roots and cause severe back and leg pain, or even cauda equina syndrome (see p. 109).

The narrowing may be congenital, or it could be due to degenerative changes, or to one vertebra slipping forward on to another (that's called spondylolisthesis).

The initial treatment is likely to be with drugs, such as anti-inflammatories – but this may not provide sufficient relief. Fortunately, spinal stenosis can be cured surgically these days. As you can imagine, the object of the operation is generally to widen the spinal canal, and so relieve the pressure on the nerve roots.

Sometimes, the 'op' can be done by using a keyhole surgery technique.

Tumours

I'm afraid that this isn't going to be a very cheery section. Unfortunately, spinal tumours (i.e. cancers) do sometimes cause back pain, particularly among the elderly. What generally happens is that a *primary* tumour develops elsewhere in the body, and then *secondary* deposits occur in the spine.

Common primary growths that can often cause spinal 'secondaries' are those of lung cancer, breast cancer and prostate cancer.

So when a person who is in the second half of life suddenly develops unexplained back pain, together with being run down or losing weight, plus perhaps the symptoms of a primary cancer somewhere, then alarm bells start ringing.

But if you have a hypochondriac streak, do please bear in mind that only a tiny proportion of cases of backache are caused by malignancy.

Summing up

Most cases of back pain are caused by simple mechanical disorders, though about 5 per cent or less are caused by disc problems (see Chapter 10). A still lower percentage is caused by really serious conditions.

However, if you ever develop any of the 'Red Flag' symptoms mentioned in Chapter 5, you should see a doctor immediately.

13

'Core strength' and exercise

As we've seen throughout this book, exercise is generally a very good thing for people who have backache. Subject to what your medical adviser tells you, it's likely that if you exercise, you'll get better more quickly.

What sort of exercise?

What sort of exercise? Well, once again subject to your doctor or health professional's advice, the following are usually excellent:

- swimming and splashing about in a pool (but avoid the breaststroke, which puts strain on the upper spine);
- walking briskly;
- jogging on grass or a 'bouncy' track (but not on a hard surface, such as a road);
- tennis and other racquet sports;
- dancing – even if it's on your own;
- aerobics;
- working out in a gym, using a programme from a qualified trainer.

I'm not going to suggest *specific* 'gym-type' exercises for you in this book, because they might not be suitable for your particular case. It's better if you do exercises that have been prescribed for you personally by your physiotherapist, chiropractor or osteopath.

Core strength

However, I would say that for most people it's a good idea to go in for what are called 'core strength exercises'. Indeed, in the twenty-first century, the phrase 'core strength' has suddenly become quite fashionable. What does it mean?

Well, in exercise jargon, your core muscles are the ones in your trunk, including the muscles around your backbone, and also the ones around your abdomen. If you've ever walked past a butcher's shop and looked at the carcasses hanging up, you'll notice that each of these poor old animals had a lot of big, powerful brown musculature around the region of the spine.

Ideally, we should have the same. But in human beings, these muscles often get rather weak and wasted – particularly if they aren't exercised regularly. However, we need them to be in good condition, so as to provide strong support for our spines. If they're floppy and lax, it's very easy for things to go wrong with the backbone. That's one reason why 'couch potatoes' are so likely to develop backache.

In an important paper published in the *Journal of Occupational Medicine and Toxicology* during 2007, W. F. Peate from the University of Arizona and his colleagues reported that getting firefighters to do regular core strength exercises reduced their annual total of back and other injuries by 42 per cent.

So your health professional may well suggest that you should do core strength exercises to build up the back muscles, and all the muscles of the torso, and also to improve the co-ordination of these muscles.

Be guided by her as to what sort of gym work you should do. She may suggest that you put yourself in the hands of a qualified instructor or personal trainer for a few weeks. Among other activities, instructors tend to encourage clients to go in for exercises with 'medicine balls', in order to improve core strength.

For instance, they commonly recommend the 'superhero' position, which is shown in Figure 13.1. The idea is that you lie on the medicine ball face-down, and contract your back muscles so that your chest and arms are parallel with the ground. This is supposed to look like a super-hero flying ...

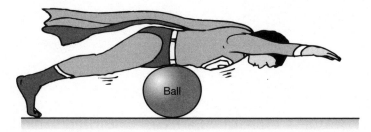

Figure 13.1 The 'superhero' core strength exercise

Another good core exercise is the 'medicine ball squat', shown in Figure 13.2. Here the idea is that, standing, you hold the ball against the wall with your upper back, and then repeatedly bend and straighten your knees while keeping the medicine ball between your spine and the wall.

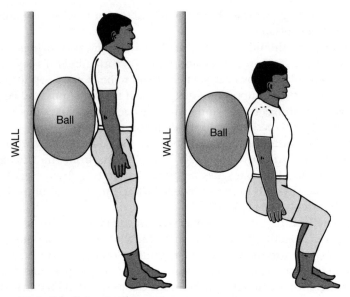

Figure 13.2 'Medicine ball squat'

Please bear in mind that pilates – and even ballet and maybe yoga – can also be good for building up core strength, along with many other types of exercise in which the back muscles are used.

Warning: If any exercise, in a gym or elsewhere, causes you back pain, then stop it immediately – even if your instructor wants you to continue!

14

Guidelines on backache

From time to time, various official bodies issue guidelines on how backache should be managed. This is quite a good thing, because – as you've seen in this book – there are all sorts of different ways of treating back pain, and some of them have very little scientific justification.

If your backache isn't responding to treatment, then it is worthwhile reading through these guidelines to see if your case is being managed in accordance with them.

If it isn't, then talk to your GP or whoever you are being treated by.

RCGP (Royal College of General Practitioners) guidelines

In the UK, the most influential set of guidelines in recent years has been the 1996 advice issued by the Royal College of General Practitioners. Though they relate to pain in the lower back, which is the most common type, much of what the guidelines say is applicable to pain anywhere in the back.

I would just say that these guidelines do have just a tiny hint of the 'Get back to work, you skivers!' attitude which is occasionally seen among doctors. My own view is that if your back is hurting you a lot, you shouldn't let yourself be pressurized into returning to the sort of work – like heavy lifting – that might make it worse.

The RCGP guidelines document is quite long, but here is my summary of the essentials:

1 If you have any 'Red Flag' (danger) signs, then you should be referred promptly to a specialist. These 'Red Flag' symptoms are listed in Chapter 5.
2 Initially, your medication should be paracetamol and/or non-steroidal anti-inflammatory agents (NSAIDs).
3 Bed rest is not generally effective as a treatment, and may make things worse. (However, can I add that this doesn't mean that you can't go to bed for a few hours – particularly on the first day of pain.)

4 It is a good idea to try to resume normal activities as soon as possible – subject to the limitations imposed by pain. (To which I would add: please don't do anything that hurts you.)

5 It is generally a good plan to return to work, but 'manual handling may be an issue'. (Again, I would like to add my own personal view – which is that if your work involves humping 100 kg bags of cement around, you should certainly think hard about the possibility of looking for another job!)

6 'Adjunct treatment' with manipulation or physiotherapy may be helpful. (This guideline is quite important, because it indicates the first admission by a major UK medical organization that osteopathy or chiropractic might be useful.)

NICE guidelines

In the UK, the views of an organization called 'NICE' have become increasingly important in the twenty-first century. The acronym 'NICE' stands for 'National Institute for Health and Clinical Excellence'.

However, please don't be misled by the title. NICE is a government-appointed body, and while it does a lot of good work in collecting and assessing medical information, the fact is that to some extent it exists in order to ration the amount of money spent on health. The authorities, though, are not very keen on admitting this.

NICE guidelines are currently being revised, but at the present time (early 2009) I would summarize the more important ones in existence as follows:

1 When treating non-specific back pain that has gone on for six weeks or more, doctors should:
   • advise people to take paracetamol;
   • consider offering short-term NSAIDs (see above) if paracetamol is ineffective;
   • bear in mind the risks of NSAIDs in older people and those (e.g. those with ulcers) who are at high risk of side-effects;
   • try to counteract the adverse effects of NSAIDs by prescribing one of the group of drugs called proton pump inhibitors (and NICE adds 'choosing the one with the lowest ... cost');
   • consider, in cases of severe pain, offering people opioid (morphine-like) drugs for short-term use;
   • try to educate people about their backs;
   • encourage a physically active lifestyle;
   • offer individual or group exercise programmes;

- consider recommending 'manual therapy including spinal manipulation of up to nine sessions over 12 weeks';
- consider acupuncture;
- consider offering a trial of tricyclic antidepressants – which, I would add, aren't in the same group as the over-used, modern, fashionable ones, like Prozac.

2 In contrast, says NICE, doctors *should not*:
- do X-rays of the lumbar spine;
- do MRIs – except when an operation is in prospect, or serious disease is suspected;
- offer injections into the back;
- offer laser therapy;
- offer interferential therapy (see Chapter 8);
- offer ultrasound;
- offer traction – because of a risk of aggravating symptoms;
- recommend lumbar supports.

To be frank, I don't know why NICE takes these uncompromising viewpoints, and why it is so against simple back-pain aids like lumbar supports – assuming they mean the cushion-like devices that London taxi-drivers put on to their seats.

However, the guidelines are currently 'up for comment' and it seems likely that they will be altered in various ways before being re-issued in the very near future.

The American Medical Association

The *Journal of the American Medical Association* recently issued the following simple guidelines for preventing back pain:

- take regular exercise;
- stretch before exercising;
- do exercises to strengthen the back muscles and make them more flexible;
- do exercises to strengthen the abdominal muscles;
- always keep a good posture when standing and sitting;
- avoid standing or being in one position for a long period;
- lose weight if you are overweight.

They've also issued the following suggestions for actually easing back pain:

- Take short periods of rest, lying flat on your back, with your knees raised by a pillow.

- Avoid long periods of bed rest, which may weaken the muscles and increase the time to recover.
- Take gentle exercise and lighter-than-normal activities.
- Take non-prescription pain-relievers and/or anti-inflammatory medications, following the manufacturer's instructions.

European Back Pain Guidelines

Several years ago, the European Commission set up a body charged with laying down guidelines on back pain for doctors and others. I would summarize the main ones they gave as follows:

- Patients should have diagnostic triage (sorting) to exclude serious spine disease and nerve root pain.
- They should be reassured that back pain is usually not serious, and that rapid recovery is expected in most people.
- They should be advised to remain as active as possible, and to return soon to normal activities.
- Psychological and social factors should be assessed.
- X-rays are not recommended, unless a specific cause is strongly suspected.
- If there are symptoms of nerve root problems, disc disorders or cancer, then an MRI is the best option.
- A straightforward X-ray is the best option for structural deformities (these are quite rare today).
- Patients should be reassessed if pain worsens, or does not resolve within several weeks.
- Serious illness should be excluded by looking out for 'Red Flag' symptoms (see Chapter 5).
- The following are 'likely to be beneficial' in various types of back pain: multidisciplinary treatment programmes, exercise therapy, spinal manipulation, pain-killers (including NSAIDs), acupuncture, behavioural therapy.

BackCare

Very good general advice and guidelines about backache can be obtained from BackCare ('The Charity For Healthier Backs').

For well over 30 years, this organization – previously known as 'The National Back Pain Association' – has been doing great work in the UK on behalf of those with backache.

Anyone who has significant back pain would derive benefit from consulting the many different pages of helpful information on their website, which is: <www.backcare.org.uk>.

Useful addresses

AECC Chiropractic College
(The Anglo-European College of
Chiropractic)
13–15 Parkwood Road
Bournemouth BH5 2DF
Tel.: 01202 436200
Website: www.aecc.ac.uk

BackCare (formerly the **National
Back Pain Association**)
16 Elmtree Road
Teddington TW11 8ST
Tel.: 020 8977 5474 (admin); 0845
130 2704 (helpline); office open
9 a.m. to 4.30 p.m., Monday to
Thursday
Website: www.backcare.org.uk

British Chiropractic Association
59 Castle Street
Reading
Berkshire RG1 7SN
Tel.: 0118 950 5950
Website: www.chiropractic-uk.co.uk

British Pain Society
Third Floor, Churchill House
London WC1R 4SG
Tel.: 020 7269 7840
Website: www.britishpainsociety.
org

**Chartered Society of
Physiotherapy**
14 Bedford Row
London WC1R 4ED
Tel.: 020 7306 6666
Website: www.csp.org.uk

General Chiropractic Council
44 Wicklow Street
London WC1X 9HL
Tel.: 020 7713 5155
Website: www.gcc-uk.org

General Medical Council
Regent's Place
350 Euston Road
London NW1 3JN
Tel.: 020 7189 5404
Website: www.gmc-uk.org
There are also offices in Belfast,
Cardiff, Edinburgh and Manchester.

General Osteopathic Council
176 Tower Bridge Road
London SE1 3LU
Tel.: 020 7357 6655
Website: www.osteopathy.org.uk

**McTimoney Chiropractic
Association**
Wallingford
Oxon OX10 8DJ

**McTimoney College of
Chiropractic**
1 Kimber Road
Abingdon
Oxfordshire OX14 1SG
Tel.: 01235 523336
Website: www.mctimoney-college.
ac.uk

**National Ankylosing Spondylitis
Society**
RCN 272258
Unit 0.2, One Victoria Villas
Richmond
Surrey TW9 2GW
Tel.: 020 8948 9117
Website: www.nass.co.uk

National Osteoporosis Society
Camerton
Bath BA2 0PJ
Tel.: 01761 471771/0845 130 3076
Helpline: 0845 450 0230 (9 a.m. to
5 p.m., Monday to Friday)
Website: www.nos.org.uk

Spinal Injuries Association
SIA House
2 Trueman Place
Oldbrook
Milton Keynes
MK6 2HH
Tel.: 0845 678 6633
Freephone Advice Line: 0800 980
0501 (9.30 a.m. to 4.30 p.m.,
Monday to Friday)
Website: www.spinal.co.uk

Welsh Institute of Chiropractic
University of Glamorgan
Pontypridd
Mid-Glamorgan
CF37 1DL
Tel.: 0800 716 925
Website: http://hesas.glam.ac.uk/
facilities/chiropractic

Index